Children with cerebral palsy

A manual for therapists, parents and community workers

Second edition

ARCHIE HINCHCLIFFE

Illustrations by Barbara Lynne Price and Clare Rogers

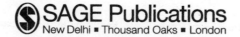
SAGE Publications
New Delhi ▪ Thousand Oaks ▪ London

First published in 2003 by Vistaar Publications
This revised second edition published in 2007 by

SAGE Publications India Pvt Ltd
B1/I-1, Mohan Cooperative Industrial Area
Mathura Road
New Delhi 110 044
www.sagepub.in

SAGE Publications Inc
2455 Teller Road
Thousand Oaks, California 91320

SAGE Publications Ltd
1 Oliver's Yard, 55 City Road
London EC1Y 1SP

Published by Vivek Mehra for SAGE Publications India Pvt Ltd, typeset in 11/13 Berkeley by Star Compugraphics Private Limited, Delhi, and printed at Chaman Enterprises, New Delhi.

Fourth Printing 2009

Library of Congress Cataloging-in-Publication Data

Hinchcliffe, Archie.
    Children with cerebral palsy: a manual for therapists, parents and community workers/Archie Hinchcliffe; illustrations by Barbara Lynne Price and Clare Rogers.—2nd ed.
        p. cm.
    Includes bibliographical references and index.
1. Cerebral palsy—Treatment.   2. Cerebral palsied children—Care.   I. Title.
    [DNLM: 1. Cerebral Palsy.   2. Cerebral Palsy—therapy.   3. Child. WS 342
H659c 2007]

RJ496.C4H565   618.92'83606—dc22   2007   2006034191

ISBN: 978-0-7619-3560-5 (PB)   978-81-7829-720-0 (India-PB)

SAGE Production Team: Rrishi Raote, Rajib Chatterjee and Santosh Rawat

To those children with cerebral palsy and their families,
and to the therapists and community workers
that I have been privileged to know

Contents

Acknowledgements
9

Introduction
10

Chapter 1
What is cerebral palsy and how does it affect children?
13

Chapter 2
Assessing a child with cerebral palsy
I. Observing and handling
25

Chapter 3
Assessing a child with cerebral palsy
II. Analysis of observations
50

Chapter 4
Contractures and deformities
71

Chapter 5
Principles of treatment
88

Chapter 6
Child, family and therapist working as a team
119

Chapter 7
Useful equipment at a treatment centre and at home
141

Chapter 8
Sensory integration problems in
children with cerebral palsy
ANNIE BROZAITIS
172

Chapter 9
Assessment and management of
eating and drinking difficulties
MARIAN BROWNE
201

Appendix A
How to make equipment from appropriate
paper-based technology (APT)
JEAN WESTMACOTT
228

Appendix B
Choosing appropriate play activities to engage
a child's active involvement in therapy
241

Glossary
244

Index
251

About the author
259

Acknowledgements

THIS book was written for the many physiotherapists who attended the courses I taught in different countries in Africa and the Middle East. I am indebted to them for the encouragement they have given me to write and the friendship they showed me during the courses.

In order to teach it is necessary to reflect on one's own learning, and my reflection causes me to be deeply grateful for the opportunities I have had to attend Bobath courses and study days. From these I learnt not only about cerebral palsy and the way it affects a child but also a problem-solving way of thinking. The tutors on these courses were invaluable inspirational role models.

I am also greatly indebted to the many wise and experienced mentors who guided me in the writing and the putting-together of the book. Chief among these is David Werner, who wrote *Disabled Village Children*. He took hours of painstaking trouble to check the drawings and provide thoughtful and apt advice on sections of the text. He was kind enough to say that he learnt a lot about cerebral palsy by reading the book.

During my many years of working with children with cerebral palsy, I have been blessed by coming in contact with people who have helped me to see the children more holistically and less as patients. Chris Underhill, who established Action on Disability and Development (ADD), and his Ugandan counterpart Charles Lwangwa-Ntale gave me the opportunity to understand how to link rehabilitation to the process of development as a whole. Peter Coleridge, who wrote *Disability, Liberation and Development*, and who invitied me to teach a course in Afghanistan, has also been a good friend and source of inspiration.

The book would not have been complete without the contributions of Marian Browne and Jean Westmacott and, in this second edition, Annie Brozaitis' chapter on sensory integration. I am deeply grateful to all three of them for the effort they put into writing these sections of the book. I would also like to thank Lynne Price for her gifted work on the drawings and Ann Sinclair and Clare Rogers for the work they did on updating these drawings and creating new ones.

Without the help and support of my husband, Peter, this book would certainly never have been written. In all our postings abroad, he made sure that my work with children took precedence over my duties as a diplomatic wife and he has constantly encouraged me in the writing of this book.

Finally I want to thank my daughter, Clare, who took great trouble to sort out a tangle I had made in chapters 2 and 3. With clinical incisiveness, she took the strands of the tangle apart and the words fell into clear, understandable sentences. She did the same for Annie Brozaitis in the new chapter. What a wonderful gift!

Introduction

THIS book has been written with therapists in mind. It is written for those therapists I worked with and who attended courses that I conducted in the Middle East, Afghanistan and Africa. But I hope that community workers, volunteers, teachers, programme managers and parents will be able to find ideas and information in the book that will help them to understand the nature of cerebral palsy and how to help children affected by it.

During the time that I lived in the Middle East and Africa, huge changes took place in attitudes to the provision of services to children with disabilities. In the seventies, funding agencies were supporting hospital-based programmes and institutional care. At this time considerable amounts of aid money were spent on training physiotherapists (never occupational therapists or speech and language therapists). This approach to rehabilitation (the medical model) was seen to fail when it was realised that so very few children could benefit from it. Even those few children who learnt to walk with aids and who received education during their time in the institutions could not easily be integrated back into their communities.

This failure and a powerful move by organisations of disabled people led to the development of the social model and the switch of donor funding to community-based rehabilitation (CBR) programmes.

There is no doubt that CBR and the philosophy behind it have achieved huge benefits for children and their families. The programmes, when they work well, mobilise the whole community so that the child and his or her family become accepted and supported by that community. Ownership and responsibility for the success of the programme is with the people on the ground. This was a very attractive idea for donors and, unfortunately, many of them thought that this would be a cheap way of dealing with a problem that otherwise seemed like a bottomless pit. This short-term view did not take into account the fact that it is not enough that people with disabilities should be accepted by their communities. Expertise must also be made available to them to enable them to be as independent as possible and, especially in the case of children with cerebral palsy (CP), this means good therapy and early intervention.

Nowadays this need is recognised—but while the idea of CBR was being promoted and developed, therapists' training programmes were being starved of support. Very few new training centres were established and those already running were pathetically underfunded. Curricula and training material could not be renewed and morale dropped very low. In all the countries where I lived and worked, therapists were given almost no teaching about paediatrics in their basic training. They had no models of good practice to aspire to and there were almost no continuing education courses at all.

The aim of the courses I ran was to start bridging the gap between the good expertise of the West and the learning needs of therapists in developing countries. Western expertise in this field does not have to be high-tech. It depends on good observational and analytical skills to solve problems and good HANDLING and communication skills to treat the child and teach families to do the same. I found the biggest difficulty in bridging this gap was that therapists, doctors and programme managers in developing countries were not easily convinced that such a seemingly simple approach could work. In the Middle East in particular, where many doctors of physical medicine were trained in former Eastern bloc countries and believed in passive treatment modalities such as hot packs and electrotherapy for children with CP, there is still a huge reluctance to consider other approaches. On the other hand, guardians of standards in Western countries responsible for course certification and validation were understandably reluctant to make adaptations to curricula and criteria for participating in their courses. This was because they did not want to be accused of watering down their standards either academically or in the level of skill acquisition. But without changes to entry criteria it is almost impossible for therapists from developing countries to get onto even the first rung of the ladder leading to internationally recognised training and ongoing education. Without adapted to curricula the courses will not prepare therapists in developing countries, either clinically or operationally, to work in their own environments.

It is my belief that the need for rigorous training programmes for therapists in developing countries is overwhelming. It is in these countries that the majority of children with CP are found. It is also in these countries that therapists need the best possible training. But they will have to work in a different way to therapists in the West because there will never be enough resources for programmes to employ therapists at a ratio of more than one therapist for every hundred children. To work effectively in these circumstances a therapist can only assess a child, plan a programme and then teach the programme to family members and community workers to carry out. There need be no watering down of standards in courses that prepare therapists to work in this way, just a change of emphasis.

The aim of this book is to be a resource for therapists. It will benefit mostly those therapists who have done a practical course. My hope is that it will give a structure within which those people responsible for children with cerebral palsy can plan an effective and feasible programme for them. This structure will reflect the complexities of the haphazard nature of the damage that cerebral palsy causes to the CENTRAL NERVOUS SYSTEM of a developing child. It also takes into account that many of the people working with these children have not had opportunities to learn how to observe children's movement and POSTURE, nor to analyse how CP interferes with these.

The structure of the book leads the reader through the process of assessing a child, planning a treatment programme and working with the family. The first chapter gives some theoretical background covering the development of normal movement, the way CP interferes with this and what possibilities there are to help the child overcome this interference. The second chapter is devoted entirely to observing, handling and finding out about a child in a holistic way. It encourages the reader to take note of every detail of the child's behaviour and performance. Not until the third chapter is the reader encouraged to analyse what it is that he has seen and taken note of. My idea was to break down into two separate operations the process of observation and that of analysis. The fourth chapter looks at the recognition of present or threatening contractures and deformities and some ideas on prevention. In the fifth chapter I have tried to condense, into what is really much too small a space, the principles of treatment of the different kinds of CP.

I know from my teaching that most people learn about principles from being given practical examples of how each principle can be applied. The danger with putting these examples in a book is that readers may think the examples are rigid treatment plans. This couldn't be further from the truth. I ask readers to use the examples only as illustrations of *one way* in which the particular principle being explained may be applied.

The sixth chapter deals with working with families, and the seventh with the equipment that can be useful both in therapy centres and for families to have at home.

The eighth chapter in this second edition is written by an occupational therapist, Annie Brozaitis. She is Bobath-trained but has also completed courses in sensory integration and has amalgamated these two approaches in her practice. She brings a new way of looking at the problems that altered sensory processing brings to a significant number of children with cerebral palsy, and imaginative ideas for helping them.

Unfortunately, in most developing countries there are very, very few speech and language therapists and a huge need for their expertise to be made available. That is why the eighth chapter, by Marian Browne, is devoted entirely to ways of helping children with CP with eating and drinking. So many children with CP in developing countries suffer desperately from not being able to take food into their mouths, manipulate it and swallow without choking that, for many mothers, nourishing their children is their overriding concern. Marian Browne is a speech and language therapist and a Bobath tutor. She worked for several years at the Bobath Centre in London.

In my own practice I have always used the Bobath or Neuro-Developmental Therapy (NDT) Approach. My aim is to demonstrate the benefits and effectiveness of the Approach and to teach the underlying skills of problem-solving and handling that lay the foundation for therapists to participate later in fully-accredited Bobath/NDT courses. Much of what I have written on the features of different kinds of CP and the principles of treatment come from the eight-week Bobath course. But this book cannot be considered as an official exponent of the Bobath Approach. It is only a reflection of the way in which I myself have interpreted the Approach and used it in the countries where I have worked. I would like to state here my indebtedness to the Bobath tutors who have helped and encouraged me over many years and to apologise to them if I have misrepresented the Bobath Concept in any way.

Throughout this book I have used 'he' and 'she' alternately when referring to children. The same is true of therapists. I hope that readers will be able to understand, from the context, which I intend.

Chapter 1

What is cerebral palsy and how does it affect children?

CEREBRAL means 'concerning the brain' and palsy means paralysis or the inability to move. CP, then, is a kind of paralysis that results from damage to the brain. The modern definition of CP is this: A persistent, but not unchanging disorder of movement and posture due to a non-progressive disorder of the immature brain (that is, under about 2 years of age).

In other words, the damage that has been done to the child's brain cannot be cured, nor will it worsen. It is 'persistent' and non-progressive. The disorder of movement and posture can, however, change. A child with CP, like all children, will grow and develop. The growth alone will make the child's ability to function more difficult because of the extra weight and length of limbs and body. So, as the child grows, the effect of the damage of the brain will be worse if the child is not helped to function as well as possible. The child's need and determination to function and interact with the world around will be strong no matter how severe his brain damage. But just making the effort to sit, stand or walk is likely to lead to the appearance of signs of CP such as SPASTICITY* or CONTRACTURES. Good intervention in the early months of a child's life will be able to channel the child's own efforts and determination into ways of moving and functioning that will minimise the effects of CP. If, on the other hand, the diagnosis is not made until the child is already showing spasticity and contractures, valuable time has been lost, perhaps irretrievably.

Good intervention is important, but so too is the child's health and family situation. The disabling effects of CP may be worse in a child who lives in poverty with few opportunities and little access to professional help.

---

* All words thus capitalised are explained in the Glossary.

It is important to realise what is meant by damage to an immature brain. A normal baby shows a huge variety of PATTERNS OF MOVEMENT early in pregnancy. Once born, and out of the fluid environment of the uterus, the baby has to learn to control and coordinate movement against the influence of gravity. He must learn to balance and, if he is in a safe and stimulating environment, he will learn to reach out and grasp. He will also learn to use his arms and legs for support and to move from one position to another. He learns this by trial and error while his brain records the sensation of movements and POSTURES. In this way, the part of his brain that controls movement and posture matures.

A baby with CP may have been damaged early in pregnancy, and may therefore have abnormal movements even before birth. He too wants to learn to balance and reach, push up and move, but can only succeed in abnormal ways. His patterns of movement do not show the great variety of the normal baby's. He may have only a limited number and these will probably not include useful ones such as weight-bearing, reaching and grasping. Because he only experiences moving in abnormal ways, his brain cannot build up a memory store of good movement experiences that allows him to develop ROTATION, SELECTIVE MOVEMENT and FINE MOTOR CONTROL.

Since CP affects a child's ability to learn to move, it is necessary to understand first how a normal child learns to hold postures and to move.

There is no space here to describe all the work that has been done, and the new laboratory techniques used, to arrive at current theories on how movement is controlled and coordinated by the brain and spinal cord. There are good neurophysiology books written on this subject, some by therapists in the field, and this work has important implications for our understanding of how to treat and manage children with CP.

The old theories held that clearly defined areas of the brain respond to stimuli from outside to produce predictable movements largely dependent on REFLEXES. More recent thinking recognises far greater complexity and interconnection between the different parts of the central nervous system and also far more possibility for adaptability and change. This possibility for adaptation and change is called plasticity.

As mentioned earlier in this chapter, the normal brain develops its ability to control movement as a result largely of its adaptability to the child's experience of postures and movements. An important additional aspect is that the necessary changes that happen in muscles, TENDONS and other peripheral structures during movement also depend on active experience of movement. An example is the child who learns to ride a bicycle at an early age: the brain will respond and adapt its pathways and connections to reflect this practice. But the particular muscles required for BALANCE and control and the tendons and other structures surrounding them will also show changes as a result of being frequently used this way. We all know that practice makes perfect. We also know that motivation, health, opportunity, encouragement and a basic talent are all important to learning the coordinated motor skills needed.

When that part of the brain that affects the ability to move is damaged, plasticity will still allow the brain to adapt, but it can only adapt to the experience of postures and movement that the child is given. If the child with CP remains lying on her back and is dressed and fed by others, that is the kind of movement her brain, and also her muscles and joints will respond to, and learning other positions and activities will be neglected. Even if the child does have treatment, if that treatment consists of passive movements for the child and the child is not actively involved, it will not bring about plasticity to the brain and will not therefore bring about changes in the way the child functions. In treatment, the child needs to be encouraged, helped and given the opportunity to move actively in more efficient, varied ways.

CHARACTERISTICS OF POSTURAL TONE IN CP

The key to the development of normal movement is a child's postural TONE. In a normal baby this tone, or readiness of the muscles to respond to messages from the brain, allows her to develop a range of patterns of movement from before birth. The child then learns to use these same patterns for useful activities in the presence of gravity. But the postural tone in a child with CP is altered, and without this basic readiness of the muscles to react it is difficult for the child to develop good functional skills without help.

There are different kinds of cerebral palsy, depending on the parts of the brain that have been damaged, and each kind is recognised by the way in which the child's postural tone is altered.

1. *Spasticity*: The muscles are stiff. The child moves in patterns that are not useful and in a limited way. As she tries to move, the muscles become stiffer. In such children the movement areas and pathways of the CORTEX are damaged.
2. *Athetosis*: There is movement all the time—unwanted movement or movement that is uncontrolled. The muscles may be stiff one moment and floppy the next. In such children the BASAL GANGLIA of the brain are damaged.
3. *Ataxia*: The muscles constantly quiver when the child tries to move. She may stiffen herself to overcome this. In these children the CEREBELLUM is damaged.
4. HYPOTONIA: The muscles are constantly floppy.

You will learn more about recognising the different kinds of CP in chapter 3.

Associated problems

Some children with CP have other associated problems. If the part of the brain that controls posture and movement can be damaged, then so can other parts of the brain.

- The intellectual capacity of the child may be damaged, making him slow to learn and understand.
- His hearing may be affected, in that he has difficulty processing what sounds he hears. In a child whose head keeps moving, it may be difficult for him to locate or attend to sounds.
- His sight may also be affected, in the sense that, although there may be nothing wrong with his eyes, his brain cannot perceive or understand what his eyes see.
- Perceptual problems can lead to a child becoming fearful of moving around. This is because he has difficulty grasping the ideas of such things as distance, perspective and height and can't make sense of his environment and how his body fits into it.
- Some children have difficulty processing sensation from their muscles and joints and for them it is difficult to know where their limbs are in relation to their bodies. They have to compensate by using their eyes.
- About half the children with CP also have EPILEPSY. This can take a very mild form, in which the child experiences temporary loss of awareness, or a severe form where the whole body shakes and the child loses consciousness for minutes at a time. These severe fits are damaging to the brain and it is important for the child to be given drugs that will reduce the number and severity of his fits. Drugs themselves, however, taken over years can also be damaging (phenobarbitone for example can interfere with the workings of the brain). It is helpful if there are a number of different drugs to choose from to find the best one for each child.

DIAGNOSIS

If a baby is born very prematurely and has difficulty breathing, it may be clear from the beginning that he has CP. This is also true of babies who sustain head injuries or who have MENINGITIS or ENCEPHALITIS. But in many cases, it is only when the baby does not develop normally that the doctor suspects CP. The baby may be abnormally floppy or rather stiff, and may not learn to sit up or reach out with her hands as other babies do. At this point the doctor must decide whether she has CP or whether the problem is one of a number of other conditions such as a tumour of the brain, a genetic or a progressive condition.

Some babies with learning difficulties are slow to learn to move and hold postures. They may not learn to sit alone until they are a year old or more. They may take a very long time to learn to walk. These children do not have CP unless they also show signs of abnormal postural tone and abnormal ways of moving. They will, however, benefit from therapy that will prevent them from getting stuck in each developmental stage and will encourage them to progress more quickly.

In developed countries it is possible nowadays to look at a child's brain through a computerised tomography (CT) scan, magnetic resonance (MR) imaging or ultrasound (in a very young baby). These methods allow the doctor to see which part of the brain is damaged, and if there is a tumour that needs to be removed.

In countries where sophisticated equipment is not available, it is still possible to differentiate between some of these conditions by taking careful note of the child's development and ways of moving. The problem is that this needs to be done over months and by the time the diagnosis is made, for example of a possible tumour, it may be too late to intervene through surgery.

For therapists, however, the important thing is to be able to recognise abnormal postural tone no matter what the cause in the child's brain. Once abnormal tone is recognised it can be changed during handling and treatment. Then the child, from a very young age, can be given opportunities to experience more normal postures and movements, helping his brain to mature. Even if he has a progressive condition, this handling and treatment will make his care easier and the quality of his life better.

HOW MANY CHILDREN ARE AFFECTED?

In rich countries, just over two out of every 1,000 births are of children born with CP. In countries with less sophisticated medical services, the number can be as high as one child in every 300 born. In developed countries, a significant proportion of children with CP are those that are born very prematurely. In developing countries, the very premature babies do not receive the sophisticated medical intervention needed for them to survive; at the same time, lack of good antenatal and obstetric care puts more babies at risk of being born with CP. In these countries there is also a higher risk of diseases such as encephalitis and meningitis causing brain damage in very young babies, resulting in CP and associated problems such as visual, hearing and intellectual impairments.

WHAT ARE THE CAUSES OF CP?

In some cases, the cause of the damage is known. In many others, it is not. In the pre-natal period, damage may be done to the baby's brain in the following ways:

- The baby's mother could have had an infection such as German measles, shingles or even simple flu in the early days of pregnancy.

- She might have taken some drugs without realising they could damage her baby.
- The PLACENTA might be insufficient (the placenta may be below the baby's head in the uterus, where it can easily be damaged).
- There is incompatibility between the mother's blood and the baby's (hyperbili-rubinaemia).

It used to be thought that a lack of oxygen during the actual birth was the cause of cerebral palsy, and parents often accused the doctor delivering the baby of negligence. More recently it has been discovered that although a few babies develop CP because of asphyxia during birth, for most babies the damage is more likely to have happened before birth. In these cases the delivery may be slower because the baby cannot move normally to assist in the process and this leads to the mistaken belief that the prolonged birth was the cause of the damage and not the result.

Babies that are born prematurely or are very small are susceptible to brain damage after they are born. This is because the blood vessels in the brain, especially those around the VENTRICLES, are very fragile. If these blood vessels are damaged there can be bleeding into the ventricles and these may push outwards and damage the surrounding brain tissue. A small amount of bleeding may not result in lasting damage but a large amount certainly will.

Head injury, meningitis or encephalitis during the early years of the baby's life can also cause CP.

HOW CAN THERAPY HELP?

In developed countries most children with CP will need to see a physiotherapist, an occupational therapist and a speech therapist. The physiotherapist will work with the child to help her develop good posture and movement, the occupational therapist will look more at the child's FUNCTION, VISUAL PERCEPTION and fine motor control and the speech therapist will help with eating and drinking and, of course, communication. In practice, the boundaries between these three professions become blurred and there is considerable overlap and sharing of responsibilities between them. All therapists need to see the child as a whole and make the child's need and desire to play and communicate the mainstay of their treatment pro-gramme while understanding how changes in postural tone as well as control of posture and movement may interfere. These are transdisciplinary core skills. In developing countries very often there will only be physiotherapists to treat the children, or there may be no therapists at all and the work will be done by rehabilitation workers or teachers. But it cannot be emphasised enough that whoever has responsibility for the rehabilitation of children with CP must have an understanding of how to help those children to play and to communicate.

In places where there are few therapists, it is likely that each one will have a huge caseload. With such pressure of work it is necessary to choose priorities and set clear goals. For any child, the most important thing is nutrition. Before movement and posture can be worked on, the child must be able to eat and drink safely and in sufficient quantities. Physiotherapists who find themselves working alone must therefore be able to advise a mother on how best to feed her baby (see chapter 9, on eating and drinking).

In the developed world, therapy for children with CP takes many different forms. This reflects the fact that there is no outright 'cure' for the condition. There are several different approaches that have been devised to help the child to grow and develop in the best way. In this book there is only space to describe them briefly. They are:

- *The Neuro-Developmental Therapy (NDT)* or *Bobath Approach*: This is the one most used in this book. It will be described in detail later in this chapter.
- *Conductive Education*: Aims to stimulate a developmental process, which will allow the child to be more easily integrated into normal education. It is carried out by conductors who combine physiotherapy, speech therapy and teaching in one programme. The children are selected and taught in groups and not all children are considered suitable. The programme was developed in Hungary by Dr Andreas Peto and later Dr Maria Hari in order to allow as many children with CP as possible to learn to walk and therefore to attend school.
- *Vojta Reflex Locomotion*: Václav Vojta bases his treatment theory on his observation that global patterns of movement with components of locomotion can be elicited in newborn babies. This leads him to believe that, in a child with CP, it is possible to influence the mechanism that controls body position and centre of gravity. He stimulates different points on the child's body to elicit RECIPROCAL creeping movements, which imprint new muscle patterns in the central nervous system. These can be stored and will lead to more normal spontaneous movement. Treatment is most effective when carried out on very young babies.
- *Move International Curriculum*: MOVE stands for Mobility Opportunities Via Education. The curriculum was developed in the United States to help learners with severe disabilities to sit, stand and walk. Move International is now used increasingly in Europe with children and young people, and sometimes with adults. It is *not* a therapy. It is a framework for good practice that breaks down functional motor tasks into small components so that progress can be charted and motor skills practised during other educational or leisure activities. It can be used in conjunction with other therapies.

CAN DRUGS HELP?

There are some drugs which can reduce spasticity, but in a short space of time the child becomes accustomed to them and it takes higher and higher doses to achieve the same results. As the dose increases so too do the side effects.

In developed countries there has been some success with botulinum injections into the muscles. Botulinum is a very powerful toxin and it works by suppressing the nerve supply to the muscle. It needs to be done with great expertise because of the high toxicity. It must always be done in partnership with a therapist so that the maximum benefit can be gained by the reduction in spasticity. It does not last more than six months and, although it can be repeated once or twice more, there is often no long-term carry over. This can leave the child and his family very disappointed and disheartened.

Perhaps the greatest benefit of trying BOTULINUM treatment is that it can demonstrate the effect of surgery but is not irreversible. So, if you want to know whether a child with a short Achilles tendon will collapse into FLEXION after the tendon is released, the botulinum injection will show you.

WHAT IS THE BOBATH (NDT) APPROACH AND HOW CAN IT HELP CHILDREN WITH CP?

Dr Karel Bobath and his wife Berta Bobath began working with children with CP in the 1940s and continued developing their treatment concept until they retired in 1987. They said that their concept was not so much a treatment schedule as a way of thinking about how cerebral palsy can affect children. The therapist must be able to observe and analyse what it is that prevents a child from carrying out functional everyday tasks and then devise a treatment programme that will prepare the child to do them. Each child is different and each one must be analysed and may be treated in an entirely different way.

Normal postural tone is the level of tension in those groups of muscles that keep us upright when gravity would pull us down. This normal level of tension also allows us to automatically adjust our position in a coordinated way to balance and move. It is the lack of this fine-tuned COORDINATION that prevents children with cerebral palsy from moving in functional ways and holding postures against gravity.

If a child's postural tone is too high she may be able to hold a position, though she will not be able to keep her balance or move much. If is too low, or if it fluctuates between low and high, she will not be able to hold a position where gravity can influence her, but she will be able to move. However, her movements will be uncoordinated and may be involuntary.

In normal movement there is reciprocal interaction between the groups of muscles. This reciprocal interaction gives us fixation PROXIMALLY (for example in the trunk, SHOULDER GIRDLE and PELVIS) to allow for movement DISTALLY (limbs). It gives us graded control of AGONIST and ANTAGONIST: in other words, coordinated CO-CONTRACTION, for smooth timing, GRADING and direction of movement. It also gives us automatic adaptation of muscles to changes in posture.

So far, research has not been able to prove that NDT treatment can directly affect the brain. However, we know that by giving a young child experience of active new movements and postures, he will achieve functional gains that can be measured. The more these new activities are practised the easier they will be to perform. This is because new connections or SYNAPSES will be made within the brain (neuroplasticity).

Fundamental to the Bobath Approach is the awareness of how normal movement develops in a child. Each developmental milestone, such as holding the head erect or sitting alone, can only be reached after a process of practising to move in certain ways and balancing within certain postures, that gradually perfects the coordination of muscle work.

For example, a newborn cannot hold his head erect because he has not learnt to lift his head against gravity. It is only as he begins to use his eyes that he is motivated to lift his head in all positions and try to hold it steady so that he can see. In order to learn to sit alone he must go through a very long process. This starts with him being able to hold his head erect. He must then be able balance his trunk on his pelvis. This means having very efficient coordination between the flexion and EXTENSION in his trunk and hips. The extension will have become fully developed when he lay prone on the floor and reached for toys with such eagerness that his head and shoulders and even both his legs lifted off the floor. The flexion becomes fully developed through his kicking as he lies on his back and then his desire to catch hold of his toes and bring them to his mouth. Once flexion and extension are developed he will be ready to rotate in his trunk. He will gain this by long weeks spent in learning to roll from front to back and back to front on the floor in order to reach toys or move himself around. With this ability to coordinate flexion and extension and to rotate in the trunk come balance reactions. Once he can sit alone and balance without using his arms for support, the whole new experience of using his hands in sitting is opened up to him.

These examples show how treatment and handling of children with CP must take into account what elements of POSTURAL CONTROL are needed before each functional goal can be achieved. Without careful analysis of what it is that is interfering with a child's ability to achieve a motor milestone or functional goal it is not possible to plan good treatment.

HOW CAN TREATMENT BE GIVEN?

There are a few therapy centres of great excellence in some of the richer countries. These centres are a resource for teaching and research and give examples of good practice. It is not possible for every child with CP to receive treatment at such centres.

In specialist centres, therapists have time to carry out long treatment sessions with each child. During these sessions the therapist will be able to use very skilled and sensitive handling techniques to enable the child to play and be active in a satisfying way. She will also be able to teach the child's carers to carry out similar treatment at home. All of this re-quires immense dedication and not every family will feel ready or able to commit to giving so much time and effort, not only to take the child to the centre whenever needed but also to carry out the treatment at home.

For most children and their families, the ideal provision of treatment would be to have a centre of excellence close enough for them to visit once in a while with their therapist or whoever is helping them in treating their child. At this centre the child will have a very thorough assessment so that the factors interfering with her function are clearly identified. Then a feasible programme for her handling and management will be discussed with all those caring for her. If this programme has realistic, achievable goals, the family will be motivated to carry it out and to return after some months for a reassessment and a new programme.

Also, in this ideal centre, specialist doctors will see children from time to time to assess their medical needs. Those children who need medication to prevent seizures, for example, need regular monitoring, and many children need to be X-rayed and checked by orthopaedic specialists to make sure they are not in danger of hip dislocation and other DEFORMITIES. Alongside these services there will also be ORTHOTISTS to provide appropriate splints, psychologists to help families with learning disabilities and behaviour problems, perhaps a toy library to encourage interesting play, and a workshop where special equipment such as chairs or standing frames can be made.

This kind of centre can be a resource for community-based rehabilitation programmes to call upon. The role of the experts based in such a centre is to advise community workers when they need help in order to progress with a particular child. They can also monitor children's progress, particularly in the years when they are growing fast and are therefore in more danger of contractures and deformities.

When such centres are not possible because there are no highly qualified experts, there is still a good deal that can be done for children with CP by community workers or volunteers who are ready to learn and who are convinced that something worthwhile can be done.

The most important thing for any child with CP is to be given opportunities to socialise with other children in his family and in his community. To do this he needs to be placed in positions other than lying down. Community workers who have the possibility of working with carpenters, or who can make pieces of equipment for positioning children out of cardboard (Appropriate Paper-based Technology, or APT), can make a huge difference to the children they work with.

MAIN CHALLENGES FACED BY PEOPLE WORKING WITH CHILDREN WITH CP

Encouraging acceptance and hope

The fact that CP causes damage to a child's brain that cannot be reversed or cured is very hard for everyone concerned to come to terms with. The doctors, therapists, community workers and others working with the child and her family have a narrow path to walk. They must help those closest to the child to find a balance between, on the one hand, acceptance of the child as she is and, on the other, hope that she can be helped to be more independent. Without acceptance that the child's disability is part of her, like the colour of her hair or size of her nose, there will always be a sense of failure and disappointment. But acceptance does not mean resignation. Acceptance must be accompanied by hope that, despite difficulties, she can achieve some or even full independence, that she can take some or total control over her own life and that there are proven ways and means of achieving this. The challenge for the professionals working with families is to recognise that each family finds the balance between these two things in their own way. It is a process that cannot be hurried. But families can be encouraged to have realistic hope and they can be sympathetically supported as they find it within themselves to accept their child's condition.

Ensuring adequate resources

Lack of sophisticated equipment and expensive aids does not have to mean that good services cannot be provided. Children need well-designed chairs and standing frames but these can be made out of cheap materials. Local carpenters and metal workers can make good-quality pieces if they are given good designs. In many programmes, parents themselves learn to make equipment for their children out of cardboard and paper (APT). This activity gives parents a very positive view of their ability to help their own child, and they can later train other parents.

Providing ongoing training programmes

There is a great need for programmes throughout the world to train all professionals and non-professionals working with children with CP. Well-trained therapists can lift a programme up so that everyone can see good results and spread the message of realistic hope mentioned earlier. The expertise that is available in rich countries must be made available everywhere. Once the expertise is available it can be adapted and made appropriate for all the different cultures and each country can set up its own sustainable ongoing training programme. Standards can then be maintained and strong cross-cultural links forged through the exchange of ideas and sharing of information internationally.

Providing good management

Working with children with CP has to be a team effort. No one person alone can achieve good results. Good management is the key to keeping the team working well.

The manager may be a doctor or may be an administrator. The title is not important, but the role that he or she plays as a leader who respects all team members equally and inspires them to achieve good results is crucial. Managers can ensure good working conditions for team members even if the pay cannot be good, they can counsel team members who are struggling and acknowledge good work, they can manage resources efficiently and they can represent the work of the programme to the outside world. Most of all, a good manager sees the work of the programme as a whole within the context of the community, and ensures that the best possible service is provided within the constraints of available resources. This can only be done by being very close to all the team members and parents and listening and empathising with their views and concerns.

Chapter 2

Assessing a child with cerebral palsy
I. Observing and handling

THE assessment of a child with CP is the key to good treatment. Each child with CP is different, and the therapist treating the child must be able to find the underlying causes of his or her inability to function normally before the treatment can be effective.

To give an example: a child with spastic QUADRIPLEGIA can sit alone on the floor when placed but her balance reactions seem not to be reliable and she is fearful of falling. It might seem reasonable, in this case, for the therapist to work to develop better balance reactions, but in fact this will not succeed unless the spasticity around the child's hips and pelvis is first reduced. A good assessment would reveal that this spasticity is the cause of the child's inability to learn to balance well.

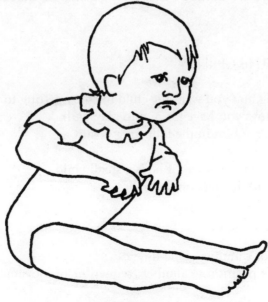

Figure 2.1
This little girl can sit alone on the floor but the spasticity in her hips prevents her
from balancing and from being able to use her hands to play

I have devoted two chapters in this short book to assessment because it is so important and because there are so many things to consider and to understand if you are to do a good job.

Each assessment needs to be broken down into three steps.

- *First*: Learn about the child through observation and handling and through listening to the family's account of how the child functions at home.
- *Second*: Analyse your observations and the information you have learnt from the family and create a full written record. During the course of this process you will decide on which type of CP the child has, in what way his postural tone is abnormal, how he compensates for this and which abnormal patterns he mostly uses to function.
- *Third*: Conclude your analysis by working out what main problems are preventing the child from being able to function well. This will provide the foundation for an effective treatment plan.

In this chapter I will describe how to gather the information needed, giving you a step-by-step guide to observing and handling the child you are assessing. In a later chapter I will deal with working with families, but obviously at the same time as you are observing and handling the child you will be learning from his family about how he is at home and how they manage.

The second and third steps of the assessment—the analysis and conclusions—I will deal with in chapter 3.

OBSERVATION OF THE CHILD

While you are observing him you want the child to enjoy getting to know you and perhaps to be interested in the toys you have for him to play with.

You will want to observe him in the following positions:

- Sitting on family member's knee (if he is a small child).
- Sitting on a stool with his feet on the floor.
- Sitting on the floor.
- SUPINE on the floor.
- PRONE on the floor.
- Held in standing (or standing alone if he can).
- Changing from one position to another (sequences of movement).

In all these positions you will be watching the child to see:

- *How much support he needs*. Take note of where the family member places his or her hands on the child. Does the child's head need support all the time? If the trunk is supported can the child support his head alone? The family member's support of the child or lack of support will tell you a good deal about the child's abilities to move and maintain postures against gravity.

- *How much movement there is.* Is it too much or too little? Normal young children who are in a wakeful state are constantly moving, but in a way that leads to more functional and purposeful activities, as they experiment and explore their environment. A child with spasticity or a child with very low tone will not show this kind of movement. His movement may be laboured or even absent. Then there are the children whose movement is too much and this interferes with their ability to come up against gravity and to hold a position. There are also some children who can move, but because of sensory or perceptual problems become distressed and fearful when they are moved or attempt to move on their own.

- *The quality of movement.* Is it normally smooth and appropriate for the child's age? Or is it jerky and in uncoordinated non-functional patterns? Is it slow and laboured and limited in its range? Is there a twisting pattern that is not normal? Is there an intention tremor when the child attempts a function?

- *What abilities (function) the child has, regardless of whether he carries them out in an abnormal way or not.* By function we mean the child's ability to carry out activities that are appropriate for his age that allow him to play and explore his environment as he wants. In order to do this he will need to be able to hold himself and to move in a number of different positions such as sitting alone or bearing weight on his legs in standing. Does he have balance reactions and PROTECTIVE RESPONSES?

- *What PATHOLOGICAL symptoms are seen.* These could be:

  1. Involuntary movements: Movements that occur when the child does not intend them.
  2. ASYMMETRY: When the movement and position of the head influences one side of the body to work in a different way to the other.
  3. STEREOTYPED abnormal patterns of movement: If these are constantly used and if they are seen with an abnormal quality of postural tone, they are certainly pathological.
  4. MORO REACTION (see Figure 2.2), or frequent STARTLE RESPONSES.

- *How the child behaves.* You will need to record how fearful the child is of strangers or a strange situation. Equally, you will need to record if he is interested in what is going on; whether he likes a particular book or a toy or enjoys social play more than toys. Do his responses indicate how well he is able to see and hear? Can he follow an object to all sides with his eyes? Does he turn towards a sound?

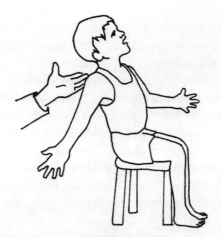

Figure 2.2
The Moro reaction occurs when a child feels his head is falling back. His arms abduct
and OUTWARDLY ROTATE, his hands and mouth open wide. He would fall if not supported

Besides these general observations there are specific things to look for and assess as the child moves or is placed in each of the following positions.

Young child sitting on family member's knee
This is usually the first position in which you will see the child. It is a chance for you to observe her while she feels secure. She will, of course, also be assessing you to see if she can trust you, so give her time before you come close to her.

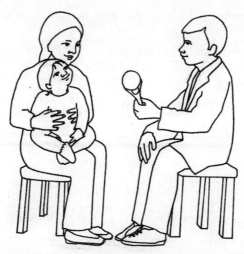

Figure 2.3
As the therapist observes the child on her mother's knee and listens to the
mother's account the child is deciding whether or not to trust the therapist

What you will want to observe in this position is:

- Does she try to hold herself upright or does she need support? Where and how does the family member give her this support?
- How much does she move? Which part of her body moves? Which part stays still?
- How much does she use her hands? If she is shy to take a toy from you, give it first to the family member and see whether the child will try to reach out for it.

While you are observing these things you can ask the family member about the child at home. Listen carefully so that you can form a clear picture, not only of what the child can do but *how* she does it. You will also want to find out how the family copes and what their feelings are about the child. Ask about:

- The medical and family history.
- Positions the child is put in at home for play, feeding, sleeping, washing, dressing and carrying.
- Difficulties with eating and drinking.
- How she communicates.
- Hearing and vision.
- The family's main problems in caring for her.

Child sitting on stool with feet flat on the floor

If the child is not able to sit alone ask the family member to show you how they would normally place her on the stool and hold her. You will want to observe in this position:

- Where the support is needed, if at all.
- Is the child's head and trunk in ALIGNMENT or is there asymmetry?
- Does she sit back on her SACRUM or can she support her trunk on her pelvis with her hips flexed at a right angle?
- Can she reach outside her BASE without losing balance—for example, reach down to the floor or out to either side?
- Does she have saving reactions?
- How well can she use her hands in this position? Does she need to use them for support or balance?

Child sitting on the floor

With the child in LONG SITTING on the floor, you should look at the following:

- Alignment of head on trunk, trunk on pelvis and pelvis on legs. Is the child sitting back on her sacrum?
- Is there head and trunk control?

- Does she balance well?
- Is her weight distributed equally on both sides?
- Do her legs adjust as she reaches out with her arms?
- Can she take weight on straightened arms?
- Can she use her hands or does she need them for support?
- Does she mostly sit with her bottom resting on the floor between her legs, which are flexed and inwardly rotated (W-sitting)?

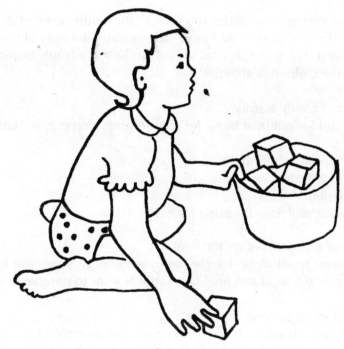

Figure 2.4
Some children find they can use their hands more easily in W-sitting

Child in supine on the floor
When the child is placed in this position you will want to observe:

- Whether the child is in alignment: Head in the middle, not pushing back into extension or turning to one side all the time, trunk straight, legs mostly symmetrical.
- What movements he makes with his head and limbs. Can he bring his hands together in front of his eyes?
- Does he kick with his legs? Is the movement symmetrical? Does he kick reciprocally?
- Can he lift his head off the floor?
- Does he try to roll?

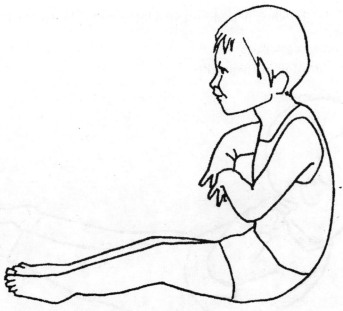

Figure 2.5
A child who cannot flex well enough at his hips when his knees are straight has to compensate with a good deal of flexion in his upper trunk. This makes his arms flex more

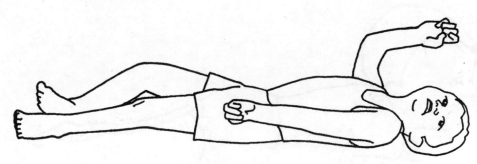

Figure 2.6
This child shows asymmetry and he is pushing back into extension

Child prone on the mat
If it is difficult to get the child into this position, or if she becomes very distressed, leave this position for a later date. If she will tolerate the position, you will want to observe:

- Can she lift her head against the pull of gravity and turn it to either side?
- Can she take weight on her forearms and reach out with either hand, or are her arms trapped under her body?

- Can she take weight when placed on extended arms? Can she push up herself onto extended arms?
- In what position are her legs?
- Are her head and trunk in alignment?

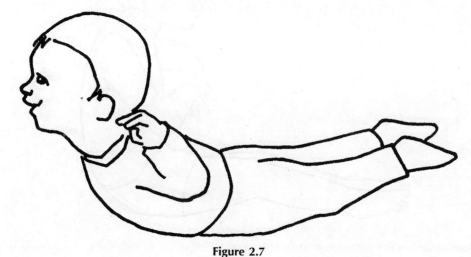

Figure 2.7
A normal baby of about 6 months can lift all limbs as well as his head and trunk against gravity

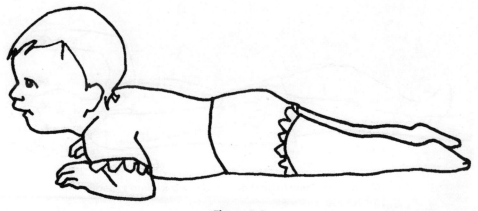

Figure 2.8
A child with spasticity in abnormal pattern of flexion in prone can only just lift her head

Child held in standing

Even if a child is totally unable to take weight on her legs, it is important for you to see what happens when she is held in standing. You, or the family member, should hold her in alignment with her hips over her feet and her knees straight. Most normal children over

7 months and most children with CP enjoy being placed in standing and respond by pushing against the ground with their feet. You will need to record if the child you are assessing does not respond like this.

You will also want to observe:

- If her legs show abnormal patterns of movement or posture.
- If she has active extension in her hips.
- If her legs collapse into flexion.
- If she has INVOLUNTARY stepping (an inability to keep both feet on the ground).

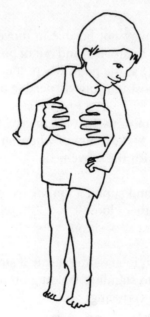

Figure 2.9
This child shows asymmetry with abnormal pattern of flexion, ADDUCTION and INWARD ROTATION of the hips and PLANTARFLEXION of the feet. The arms are in abnormal flexion, inward rotation and pronation

If a child is able to stand, perhaps holding with one or both hands, you will want to see:

- How much does she need her hands for balance or support?
- Do her feet react normally to taking her body weight?
- Does she hold with good grip?
- Does she have active extension in her hips?
- Do her knees HYPEREXTEND?

Sequences of movement

By 'sequences of movement' we mean the way the child moves from one position to another. In order to do this the child must have some of the following:

- The ability to shift weight on to one side.
- Coordinated rotation in the trunk.
- The ability to bear weight on limbs and move over them.
- Head and trunk control.
- Balance reactions.

More severely affected children may not be able to move out of any position in which they are placed. Others may be able to move in and out of positions but in an abnormal way. Still others may get stuck, especially at the point where they must come up against gravity. As you watch the child change his position you will need to observe how he is compensating for his difficulties.

The following sequences are the most useful ones for you to observe a child carrying out. As she tries to do each one you must take notice of where she is getting stuck. Help her just enough so that she can continue with the movement.

- Rolling from prone to supine and supine to prone over either side.
- Sitting up from supine over either elbow.
- Changing from sitting to CRAWLING position.
- Crawling.
- Moving from crawling position to standing, using a stool if necessary.
- Moving from sitting on stool to standing, holding on if necessary.
- Stepping sideways holding on (cruising).
- Stepping forwards with support.
- Walking with hands/hand held.
- Walking unaided.

In each sequence there are different observations to be made. We will take each of them in turn.

Rolling from prone to supine

Normal rolling from prone to supine involves being able to turn the head to one side, to shift weight onto one side, to rotate and extend the trunk, first lifting either one shoulder or one leg off the floor, then twist around the BODY AXIS in a controlled way over the arm caught underneath the body, to finally lie supine.

The child you are assessing may be able to roll from prone to supine, but not in the normal way. Usually the problem is that there is very little rotation and in order to come into supine the child must use her head to initiate total extension and flick herself over. Another child may curl into flexion and roll in one motion.

NORMAL ROLLING FROM PRONE TO SUPINE

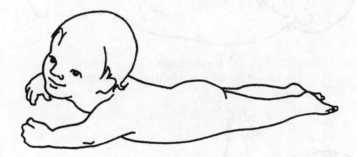

Figure 2.10a
Weight shifts onto left side

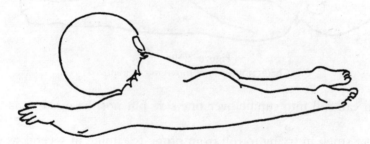

Figure 2.10b
Head and trunk extend and rotate

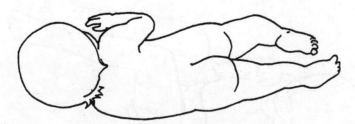

Figure 2.10c
Arm lifts up and trunk further rotates

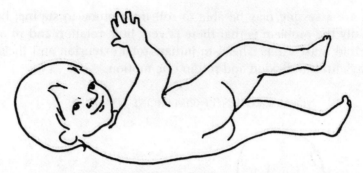

Figure 2.10d
Leg lifts off the floor and head rotates further

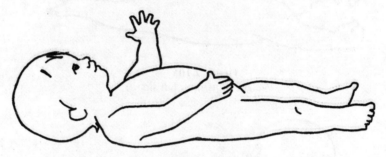

Figure 2.10e
Child controls final move into supine

Many children can roll into supine over one side but not the other. It is important to record which.

A child may get stuck in trying to roll from prone to supine in several ways, as can be seen in the following drawings.

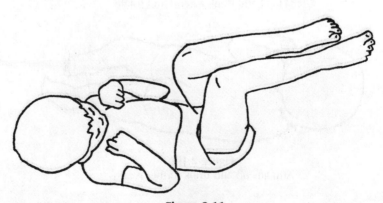

Figure 2.11
Head and shoulder girdle strongly flexed

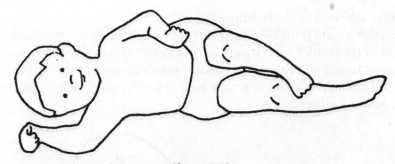

Figure 2.12
Arm trapped awkwardly when child rolls to side

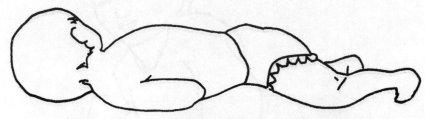

Figure 2.13
Hips strongly flexed and abducted

Rolling from supine to prone
Normally, a child will initiate rolling from supine to prone by turning her head and maybe reaching across her body with an arm. It is equally normal, though, to initiate rolling by bringing one leg across. In either case, a normal child will find herself in SIDE-LYING and from there, by lifting and turning her head, can roll into prone. In order to do this smoothly and without discomfort the child must be able to adjust the underneath arm so that it is not trapped in an awkward position. Because she is able to extend and rotate her head, trunk and hips, she will be able shift her weight off the trapped arm. A child who lies in supine with her arms widely abducted, outwardly rotated at the shoulders and flexed at the elbows cannot roll over without coming up on one elbow or causing pain at the shoulder joint.

When you ask the child you are assessing to roll over, it helps to first ask her to follow a toy with her eyes. Move the toy so that she turns her head to one side and then extends it. Show her where you are placing the toy and encourage her to roll to reach it. Watch carefully to see how she rolls over. Is it all in one piece, like a log, or does she have some rotation in her trunk? Does she sit up rather than roll into prone? Can she roll over one side only? If she can't complete the roll take careful note of her difficulties. In what part of the sequence is she getting stuck, and which part of her body is causing the problem?

Sitting up from supine over either elbow

In order to do this a child must be able to lift his head off the floor, shift his weight onto one side (rotation of the trunk), take weight on his flexed arm and push up into sitting. This sequence comes late in a normal child's motor development (at about 9 months). As you watch the child attempting to do this, take note at which point he has difficulty. Is it easier on one side than the other?

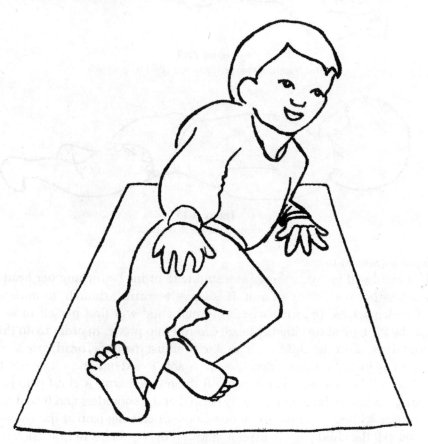

Figure 2.14
Normal coming up to sitting, with weight-bearing on one arm and rotation in trunk

Changing from sitting to crawling position

This involves the child being able to shift her weight onto one side and take the weight on both her arms on one side of her body, while maintaining her balance (MOBILE WEIGHT-BEARING). Using her arms as a pivot she then has to rotate her trunk and lift her pelvis over her flexed knees to come up into all-four kneeling. Where does she have difficulty? Is it better over one side than the other? Can she reverse the sequence and come back into sitting again?

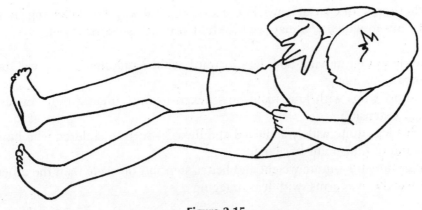

Figure 2.15
Failure to come to sitting because no weight-bearing on arm,
no rotation in trunk and not enough hip flexion

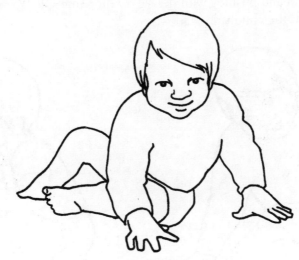

Figure 2.16
In changing from sitting to crawling, the child's arms are fully extended while her legs are flexed.
She has to balance her weight on her arms, rotate her trunk and bring her knees into
position under her hips so that they can take her weight

Crawling

Most normal children learn to move around the floor on hands and knees (crawling). In order to crawl normally a child needs rotation in her trunk and mobile weight-bearing on all her limbs to allow her to take weight on each one in turn. She also needs to be able to support herself on legs bent at right angles at hips and knees and on arms with straight elbows. Then she needs to be able to move her arms and legs reciprocally and shift her weight from side to side.

Some children with CP can crawl, but in an abnormal way. The following are some of the abnormal ways in which you may see the child you are assessing crawl:

- Bunny hopping, moving both legs forward at the same time in the way that a rabbit (bunny) hops along.
- Very short steps with knees and hips flexed to more than a right angle—not good enough extension.
- With his legs quite widely abducted and flexed—seen in children who have difficulty balancing in four-point kneeling.
- With asymmetry—more weight and better steps on one side than the other.
- Most weight over arms, with legs dragging.

Some normal children choose not to crawl, and instead move around the floor in sitting. This is called bottom shuffling. Those children with CP who are more affected on one side than the other will sometimes bottom shuffle in side-sitting. They will pull themselves along using one hand and pushing with the leg on the same side. You will need to take note of the side on which the child side sits.

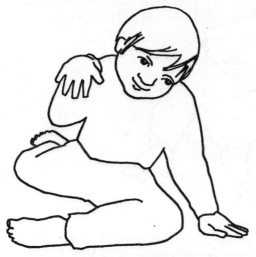

Figure 2.17
Bottom shuffling using only one side;
other side is strongly retracted

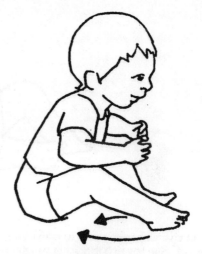

Figure 2.18
Symmetrical bottom shuffling
using a lot of flexion

Other children with CP will bottom shuffle symmetrically, but you will need to look at their sitting posture and note how they are using their legs and arms as they move around.

Pull to standing from all-four kneeling
A child will normally do this at around 9 months of age. He will come up into high kneeling by grasping the edge of a chair, for example, bring one leg forward into half kneeling and then push on the forward leg and pull with his arms to come up into standing. Most normal children will prefer to use one leg to push themselves up, either left or right, but they *can* use either leg.

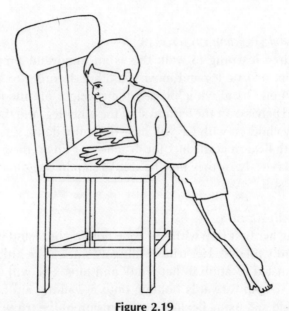

Figure 2.19
Arms strongly pulling leads to spasticity in legs. One leg is then
not able to move in a different pattern to the other

In the child you are assessing you should note in which part of the sequence and which part of the body he is having difficulty, or where he uses abnormal patterns. He may, for example, have very little DISSOCIATION between his legs and may pull them both into extension at the same time as he drags his weight up over his legs using strong flexion in his arms. He may take most of the weight on his arms and very little on his legs. He may have involuntary movements that interfere with his ability to organise the sequence.

Pull to standing from sitting on a stool
A normal child who stands up from sitting on a stool will first shift her weight forward, bringing her head almost in front of her feet. This brings her centre of gravity forward and makes it easy for her to use her legs to push up into standing. She does not need to use her hands at all.

Children with spasticity may use their arms to do the work, and pull themselves up with a good deal of flexion of their arms while the legs extend in a spastic pattern. A child with spastic diplegia may need to take steps immediately in order to keep her balance. A child with fluctuating tone may be able to stand up, but with poor balance, and he may not be able to stand still.

You should note if the child can take weight equally on both her legs as she pulls into standing.

Stepping sideways while holding on (cruising)

For all normal children learning to walk this is an important preparation because they are learning to balance on one leg and move the other. In order to be able to do this they have to hold on with one hand while placing their weight on one leg. They then have to balance the trunk and pelvis over the leg and shift the other leg, and the other hand, sideways into ABDUCTION. Many children with CP will have difficulty doing this. They may manage in an abnormal way, with flexion at the hip, for instance, or up on their toes. They may not be able to hold the pelvis steady, or they may be able to step in one direction and not the other because the pelvis is stiff.

Stepping forwards with support

A normal child taking her first step with someone holding her hand will do so with her legs abducted and outwardly rotated. Her trunk will sway sideways a little because she does not yet have fully coordinated rotation in her trunk and hips. She will waddle. Children with CP are often taught to step forwards holding onto a walking aid but they may do so by holding the pelvis rigid and using flexion and extension of the trunk to compensate for the lack of movement in the pelvis. Their steps will be small, their balance poor, and as they tire this will worsen. You may notice that they can take bigger steps with one leg than with the other.

Children who have asymmetry and involuntary movements in their arms may not be able to hold on with their hands but may be able to take steps if they are supported at the pelvis.

Walking unaided

Children with HEMIPLEGIA, moderate DIPLEGIA, mild quadriplegia and ataxia are most likely to be able to walk unaided. Many athetoid children learn to walk unaided, often at a late age. All have different problems and often the way they compensate for their difficulties may put them in danger of contractures and deformities. That is why it is important for you to observe well how the child is walking, what difficulties she has and how she is compensating for them.

The following are some of the features of a child's gait that you will need to observe:

- Are there good balance reactions and protective responses?
- Are the child's feet widely separated or close together?
- Is there equal weight distribution on both legs?
- Does the heel touch the ground first or the toes?
- Is there equal step length with both legs?
- Does the child have to move her head and trunk more than is normal to compensate for stiffness around pelvis?
- Do the child's arms get stiffer the more he walks?
- Can the child stop when asked to?
- Can the child change direction while walking?

The following are some examples of compensatory activities:

- Some children give themselves stability by holding the pelvis rigid. In order to then move and take steps, they must flex and extend the trunk in an exaggerated way.
- Other children may walk with too much flexion in their knees and hips (crouch gait). In order to keep upright they must strongly hollow their LUMBAR SPINE.
- Some with poor stability learn to stand and walk by holding their hands together. This gives them a fixed point from which to move.
- Yet others walk with their arms held up to help give them extra extension.

This completes the section on observation. Of course it is not possible to describe every detail of how a child might hold different postures and move. But I hope this section has given you some guidelines on the sort of thing you could record and use in your analysis of the child's problems.

HANDLING

Through observation we see patterns of movement and posture. We see how a child functions and how he compensates for incomplete function. But in order to find out more about the underlying causes of the problems and abnormalities that we see, we must feel with our hands the degrees of change in tension in the child's body as he moves and makes efforts to function in different postural patterns. We must also assess the range of movement in his joints by handling them.

Assessment and treatment go hand in hand. When we find stiffness, floppiness or instability it should be part of our assessment to see how easily and quickly the child can respond to changes that we make or support we give.

Postural tone

The main characteristic of CP is abnormal postural TONE. If a child's postural tone is normal, he will have enough tension and readiness in his muscles to allow him to hold himself in a wide range of positions even where gravity might cause him to fall. His normal tone will also allow him to carry out coordinated functional movements without effort. If we move one of his limbs we will find that it feels light and there is neither too little nor too much resistance to the movement. The child with normal tone helps us to move his limb smoothly.

Moving the child's body, then, is a good way for us to find out the state of tension (or the tone) in his muscles. We will want to do this in a variety of different positions and take note of when there is more or less resistance to our efforts to move the child. We will also want to see if, by positioning and handling the child in certain ways we can change the tone quality.

In sitting
While the child is sitting, alone or supported, either on the floor or on a stool, you can feel the tone in his arms and shoulder girdle.

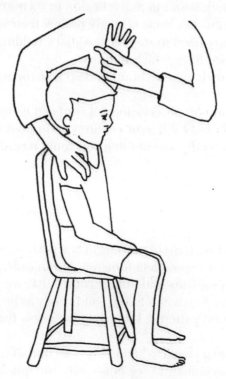

Figure 2.20
Lifting a child's arm right up helps the therapist to feel what the tension in the muscles is like

If his tone is lower than normal you will feel little resistance as you raise each arm in turn over his head with his elbow either bent or straight. You will feel his whole limb to be heavy and his joints will allow you to move his arm in a greater range than normal. His elbows may hyperextend, his wrist and fingers extend more than normal. His shoulder and shoulder girdle will feel quite loose.

We can try to change abnormally low tone by placing the child, still in sitting, so that he is bearing weight on his extended arm on a table in front of him. We can help him to bear weight on his arms by holding his elbows straight and stimulating him by talking to him or getting him to follow a toy with his eyes. The secret of good handling is then to withdraw support, even if only for a second, so that he holds the position himself. As soon as he begins to collapse your hands must be ready to support him again.

If his tone is high, when you try to move his arm you will find resistance. If his abnormal pattern is predominantly flexion, as you raise his arm you will feel that he is pulling against you into adduction and inward rotation. At the same time you may notice increased EXTENSOR TONE in his legs so that his hips extend a little and his bottom slides forward on the stool. If the abnormal pattern in his arms and trunk is predominantly extension you will probably be able to lift his arm to shoulder height, but this may put him in danger of falling backwards. You may feel resistance when you try to bring his arms down and extend his elbows.

If his tone is fluctuating, as you move the arm you may feel it to be heavy and easily moved but it may also suddenly become stiff and then floppy again. These tone changes will interfere with your efforts to move the limb smoothly.

It is part of assessment to see if we can change the way the child moves or holds postures. By changing one or two elements of the typical pattern we alter the abnormal pattern and we may be able to help the child to move more normally. This is where treatment and assessment overlap.

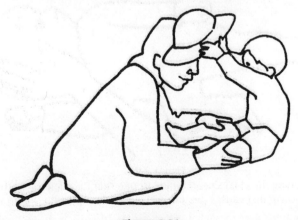

Figure 2.21
Part of assessment is trying out what happens when we change something. Here the therapist flexes and outwardly rotates the child's hips to see if it will help him to get better flexion in his hips at the same time as actively reaching forward with his arms and extending his trunk

So, briefly, during assessment, we try out some changes in the child's position to find out how he responds and also if this might improve his ability to function.

For example, a child who sits on the floor with his weight back on his sacrum, his hips somewhat extended, adducted and inwardly rotated, cannot balance well or easily use his hands. To change this we can try to keep his knees extended but abduct and outwardly rotate his hips a little. This should allow his trunk to come forward over his legs and we can help him to actively use his arms to reach up and out. If this is too difficult it may be better to try the same activity sitting on a low stool.

We want to see how well he accommodates to this kind of handling and also want to find out if the same activity would be worthwhile and feasible for a family member to do at home.

Much more about how to change and influence the child's tone will be found in chapter 5, on principles of treatment.

In supine

Try lifting his head off the mat. Do you feel resistance? Turn his head to one side and hold it there. Wait a few seconds to see if he flexes his arm and leg on the side away from his face. If he does, this shows the position of his head is influencing the movement in the rest of his body.

Move his arms slowly in all directions to feel if there is resistance. Is there, for example, spasticity in the shoulder girdle that holds his shoulders and arms in retraction and makes it difficult to bring his hands together in midline?

If he is crying and voluntarily resisting, you wait for a chance to try when he is less distressed.

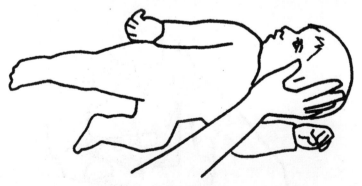

Figure 2.22
Holding the child's head turned to one side for a few seconds
will show if that causes the arm and leg on the opposite side to flex

Hold his hands and pull him slowly to sitting. If he is very floppy hold his arms at the elbows. Does his head fall back? When he is sitting, talk to him and keep eye contact with him. Slowly lower him to lying again and note at what point he can no longer prevent his head from falling back.

In prone
If the child cannot come up on his elbows, try placing him there. Notice how difficult this is. Does he seem to want to pull his arms under his body all the time? Is his tone too low around his shoulder girdle for him to hold himself up? If any of these activities in prone are too difficult, try placing him over a rolled up blanket or over your leg so that his elbows are on the ground and his chest supported. Can he tolerate this? Can he lift his head and turn it? Try getting him to use his hands to grasp a toy in this position. Is his back actively extending, even if only momentarily?

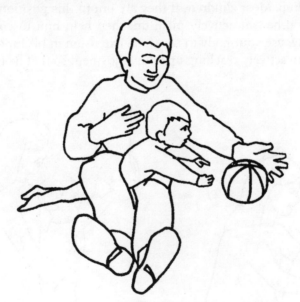

Figure 2.23
The therapist is finding out if the child can actively extend his head and trunk in prone
if he is given help. In this case his trunk is already lifted up and he has fixation on his pelvis

A child who has INTERMITTENT SPASMS is most likely to have them while he lies prone. Note if these are a problem to him (they are usually uncomfortable). You will be aware of them when his hips suddenly come up off the mat and his head pulls into flexion. If they occur, see if you can reduce them by pressing down firmly on his sacrum and rocking him very slightly from side to side.

Sequences of movement

In a small book such as this there is no room to describe how you can help a child to carry out all possible sequences of movement. The principle is to use your hands to give the child stability where he needs it in order to help him to have a fixed point from which to move. You then use KEY POINTS OF CONTROL to make it possible for him to move and change his position.

For example, if you want to help a small child to push up into standing from sitting, have him sit on your knees with his feet flat on the floor. Hold his two knees with one of your hands. Support his trunk with the other. Push down through the hand holding his knees (stability) while tipping his whole body forward so that his head is farther forward than his feet. Tell him to stand up. Most children, if they are put in this position, love to push into standing. Wait to see if he can actively push up, then help him to complete the action. When he is in standing, use your body to FACILITATE extension in his hips and hold his body in alignment. Keep him actively reaching up with enjoyment so that he is further facilitated to actively extend.

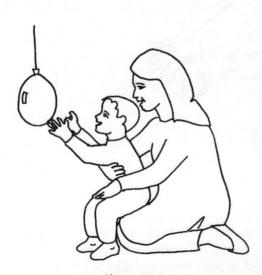

Figure 2.24
The therapist uses one hand to press down on the child's knees. With the other hand she supports his trunk and helps him to bring his head forward just in front of his feet. He will then be in a good position to try to push up into standing

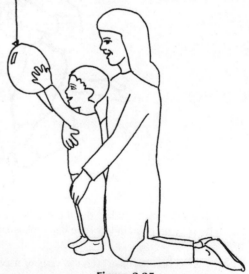

Figure 2.25
Once he has pushed up a little himself the therapist supports him with her body, making sure that his hips are in good extension and his body in alignment. She then assesses if he can actively extend his hips, knees and trunk in this position

This chapter has described all the different ways in which you can find out as much as possible about how much a child with CP can do and, equally important, how he does it. It has also given you some idea of how to find out what he might be able to do if he has the right kind of help. If your findings are detailed enough and well recorded, you will be able to analyse them and discover the underlying causes of the child's problems with posture and movement.

Chapter 3

Assessing a child with cerebral palsy
II. Analysis of observations

THIS chapter will guide you through the process of making a record of waht you have observed. The object is not just to store the information but also to analyse it, leading to an understanding of the child's problems. You could use the following headings as a framework for your report:

Diagnosis (which kind of cerebral palsy)
History
Family's concerns (see chapter 6)
General impression
Abilities
Inabilities
Basic tone
Postural patterns
Contractures and deformities
Main underlying problems

In the first section of this chapter you will learn how the different kinds of CP are classified. Matching your observations of the child you are assessing with the features of each kind of CP will help you diagnose which kind the child has. The second section deals with all the other information you need to consider, under headings that will make it easy for you to record and think about. The third section helps you to use all the information and knowledge gathered with the help of the first two sections to identify the underlying causes of the child's problems.

SECTION 1

Diagnosis (which kind of cerebral palsy)

The different types of CP can be described under two main headings: the parts of the body affected and the quality of the child's postural tone. A child whose body is totally affected is described as having quadriplegia, one whose lower limbs are mostly affected, diplegia, and one whose upper and lower limbs on one side are affected, hemiplegia.

A young child with DIPLEGIA may also show some spasticity in her arms and trunk, but these parts will be much less affected. In addition, one side of her body will be more affected than the other.

In a child with quadriplegia, his whole body will be equally affected. Although in a young child the arms and shoulder girdle often have spasticity early on, the legs may not move much and what movement there is may be like that of a very young baby. As the child gets older and tries to come up against gravity the spasticity is seen in the legs as well.

Deciding on the quality of tone is the next task. The child's tone may be described by one of the following terms:

Severe hypertonus: Stays high even at rest
Changeable hypertonus: Changes between fairly normal at rest to high with effort or
　　emotion
Fluctuating: Varies between low and high, hardly ever normal
Intermittent: Varies between low and normal
Flaccid or *hypotonic*: Stays low

A child with severe hypertonus (see HYPERTONIA) will be stiff in most positions and during all activities, often even at rest. A child with changeable hypertonus may have almost normal tone at rest, but while trying to hold positions against gravity and while using effort he may become very stiff. When the tone is fluctuating, it will vary between abnormally high and abnormally low and back again, often in a very short space of time; it will hardly ever be normal. When the tone is intermittent, it will vary between abnormally low and normal.

When you move the child's limbs through a wide range, the kind of resistance you feel will tell you what the tone is like. You can learn more by watching him move and play.

Different kinds of abnormal tone cause the features associated with different kinds of cerebral palsy. To help you decide what type of CP the child you are assessing has, look at

Features of severe spastic CP

- **Exaggerated co-contraction**
- **Tone unchanging with changing conditions**
- **Tone increased proximally more than distally**
- **Little or no movement**
- **What movement there is occurs only in middle range**
- **Difficulty in initiating movement**
- **Difficulty in adjusting to being moved or handled**
- **No balance or protective reactions**
- **Poor RIGHTING REACTIONS**
- **ASSOCIATED REACTIONS causing increased spasticity not seen as movements**

the boxes in this chapter and compare the notes you have made with the features described for each type. As you match the features with the child's you will probably be able to see what kind of cerebral palsy he has.

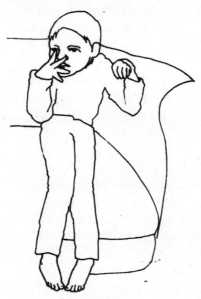

Figure 3.1
Child with severe spasticity

Severe spasticity can be seen in a child who is a quadriplegic, a diplegic or a hemiplegic.

Exaggerated co-contraction means that flexors and extensors (or agonists and antagonists) are equally spastic. So there will be resistance to moving the child's limb in any direction. When a child with severe spasticity tries to move, or when he is handled and moved, he can become very flexed or very extended.

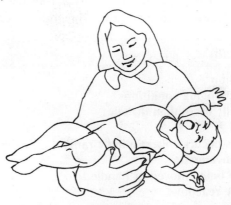

Figure 3.2
Child with severe spasticity in total extension pattern

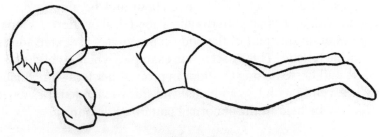

Figure 3.3
Child with severe spasticity in total flexion pattern

Features of moderate spasticity

- **Changeable hypertonus, rising from relatively normal at rest to high or very high with stimulation, effort, speech or emotion (particularly fear).**
- **Poor balance and protective responses**
- **Spasticity more distal than proximal**
- **Associated reactions, seen as movements, likely to increase spasticity as child uses effort to function**
- **Child likely to move and function using stereotyped abnormal patterns**
- **Total patterns of flexion or extension, which are likely to be compensatory—i.e., flexion in lower limbs with extension in upper and vice versa**

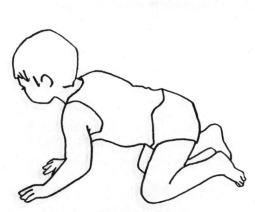

Figure 3.4
Using flexion spasticity to move

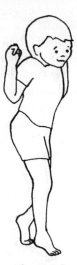

Figure 3.5
Using extension pattern to move

A child with moderate spasticity will move about and be able to do some things for himself, but mostly with abnormal patterns and a good deal of effort. Compensatory spastic patterns, where flexion in one part of the body compensates for extension in another (and vice versa) are characteristic. This is seen, for example, when a child uses flexion in her arms and trunk to pull herself along the floor in prone—her legs stiffly extend and adduct. It is also seen when a child with legs adducted and stiffly extended tries to stand—her arms and upper trunk may be held in the abnormal pattern of flexion.

There are two main types of ATHETOSIS: dystonic and choreo-athetosis.

Features of choreo-athetosis

- **Constant fluctuations in tone between abnormally high and abnormally low**
- **Involuntary movements**
- **Lack of adequate co-contraction, leading to difficulty in sustaining postural control against gravity and poor proximal fixation**
- **Inadequate balance and protective responses**
- **Asymmetry**
- **Lack of grading of movement**
- **Child dislikes being still**

Features of dystonic athetosis

- **Tone fluctuates between fairly low and very high, staying high for longer than in choreo-athetosis**
- **Lack of proximal fixation**
- **Dystonic spasms causing twisting, non-purposeful patterns that are sustained sometimes for minutes at a time**
- **Very marked asymmetry**
- **Danger of contractures and deformities such as scoliosis**
- **Older children show more spasticity and their picture can look like spastic quadriplegia**

The characteristic of a child with choreo-athetosis is that he constantly moves, but not always in a useful, functional way. He has poor stability, particularly in his head and trunk, and this lack of proximal stability allows the involuntary movements to be even more out of his control.

Some children with athetosis compensate by fixing themselves in ways such as W-sitting or hooking their feet around the legs of the chair. But a child with athetosis, unlike a child with spasticity, does know how to move. He can take steps, for example, if someone holds his trunk and pelvis steady. He will persevere to reach and grasp because he knows how to do it, lacking only a fixed base from which to move.

He also has a problem getting his head, hands and eyes to midline and holding them there. The asymmetry that is a characteristic of all athetoids is one of their most disabling features. Since the position of the head in these children often influences the postural patterns in the rest of the body, any movement of the head causes involuntary movements in all the limbs.

Lack of grading of movement means that he cannot smoothly control a movement through a range. He can shoot from full flexion in a joint to full extension.

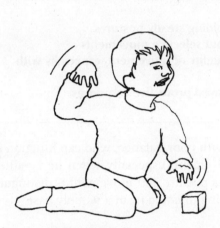

Figure 3.6
This athetoid child needs W-sitting to give him stability. He also lacks symmetry

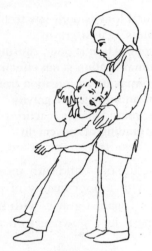

Figure 3.7
He loves to take steps but he lacks sufficient co-contraction to hold himself upright

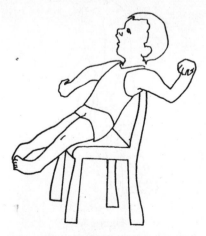

Figure 3.8
Athetoid child with dystonic spasm

The child with dystonic athetosis, on the other hand, shows sudden changes in tone either in response to his head movements or because of emotion. The pattern often involves extension of the upper trunk with rotation of head and trunk to one side and leaves the child stuck in a twisted position at the extreme end of his range of movement. This high tone can be sustained for some time before it finally drops to low as suddenly as it shot up.

Features of ataxia

- **Postural tone is fairly low to normal, and the child can move and can hold some postures against gravity**
- **Co-contraction is poor, causing difficulty in holding steady postures**
- **Proximal fixation is not effective for carrying out selective movements**
- **There may be an intention tremor and jerky quality of movement, especially with effort and up against gravity**
- **Inadequate balance reactions and slow or delayed protective responses**
- **Poor grading of movement**

The picture of a child with ATAXIA is of a child with poor balance, who can function fairly well but with a poor quality of posture and movement, especially when he is sitting or standing up against gravity with little support. His posture and movement is distinguished by shakiness, by a slowness to react and by seeming to come from a wobbly base.

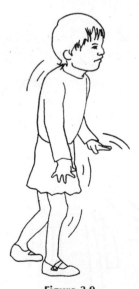

Figure 3.9
Ataxic child has poor postural control because of
intermittent tone. She also has poor balance

Features of flaccidity, or hypotonus (low tone)

- **Child takes up all available support**
- **Poor head and trunk control**
- **Child doesn't move much**
- **Joints are hypermobile (wide range of movement)**
- **Child doesn't respond even to quite strong stimulation**
- **Associated problems such as poor vision, hearing, speech and feeding are very common**

If the child has such low tone that he can hardly hold himself up against gravity, it will be easy to recognise the features described. But if his tone is not so very low you will need to recognise the same features when they are less obvious.

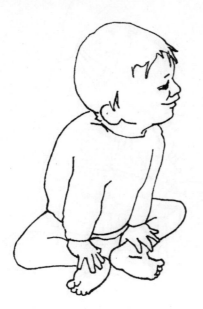

Figure 3.10
Child can't use hands to play because he needs them to support his floppy trunk

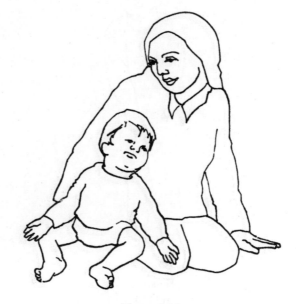

Figure 3.11
Child with very low tone:
Needs a lot of support

It is important to know that in a very young child, features of flaccidity are often only temporarily present. As the child tries to become more active the tone changes, and you may find transitory spasticity or fluctuating tone that shows itself briefly before the child becomes flaccid again.

Mixed

Children with athetosis and ataxia often also have spasticity. This may mask the involuntary movements and tremor, but these will be seen if the spasticity is reduced.

Athetoid and ataxic children are often flaccid when they are young. The features of athetosis and ataxia show themselves only when the child attempts to move.

This is a brief picture of each of the different kinds of CP. If it is possible for you to match the picture you have built up of the child you are assessing to one of these descriptions, then you can record your classification. It might, for example, be 'Moderate spastic diplegia', or 'Athetoid with spasticity'. Sometimes it is not easy to decide straight away.

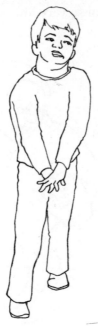

Figure 3.12
Mixed (athetosis with spasticity): This young man uses spasticity in his upper body to give him fixation

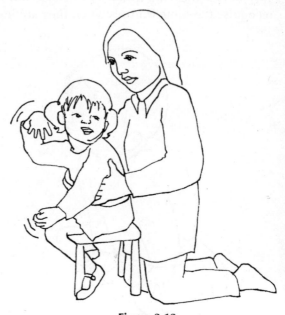

Figure 3.13
Child shows low tone in her trunk but fluctuating tone in her arms

SECTION TWO

This section describes how to record all the other information about the child under the report headings suggested at the beginning of this chapter. Family concerns are a key part of the assessment and should be recorded, but the issue of working with families needs a whole chapter to itself and will not be described here (see chapter 6).

History

Under this heading you record what you know from the medical records of the child's birth history and any following events that are relevant. This is also a good place to record any other impairments the child may have. These associated problems could include:

- Visual impairments
- Hearing impairments
- Learning problems
- Epilepsy
- Perceptual problems
- Speech problems
- Feeding problems

It may not be possible for you to find out all the additional problems the child may or may not have at the first or second meeting, but at least you should record those that you do know.

General impression

Under this heading you give a brief picture of what the child is like as a person, as opposed to a 'case'. Is she friendly or frightened, interested or unresponsive, dependent on her mother or eager to explore? Try to write down, first of all, the positive things about the child so that someone else, looking at your report, will be given the positive as well as the negative aspects of the child's condition.

There are some general personality characteristics that go with the different kinds of CP that might be useful for you to know about; but, of course, each child is an individual and it would be a mistake for you to think that, for example, every athetoid child has the same personality.

Athetoid children, in general, can show abrupt changes of mood, almost echoing changes in their postural tone. Although their constant movement makes it seem as if they have poor concentration, in reality they can show surprising persistence and determination, and this helps them to achieve a good deal. It is important for you to remember that most athetoid children have normal intelligence.

The child with spasticity, in contrast, can be fearful of moving and being moved. This leads her to dislike changes and to be unadventurous and rather passive. Some children with spasticity, however, love to be moved, but only if they feel secure with the person handling them.

Abilities

It is good to have on the first page of your assessment a clear list of things the child *can* do along with a brief description of *how* he does them for example, 'Can crawl but uses too much flexion'.

No matter how disabled a child is, he will be able to do something. Perhaps he can just turn his head or take weight on his legs when placed in standing. Perhaps he can indicate his needs by moving his hands. As long as what he does can be said to have a useful function, it is an ability, even if he uses abnormal patterns to achieve it.

In this list you should include not only those abilities that you have seen for yourself, but also those the parent tells you about. For example, a child may not be ready to show you that he can crawl, but his mother may say that he crawls everywhere at home. You must record in the notes what his mother describes and try later to see for yourself.

Inabilities

These are the functional activities that the child cannot do and which you and his family will be working towards achieving. You must think of:

- What postures he cannot maintain.
- What handling and movement he cannot tolerate.
- What hand function he does not have.
- What mobility around his environment he does not have.
- What sequences of movement he cannot achieve.

For an older child with severe spasticity and with fixed contractures, you will not mention that he cannot walk alone. You might instead say that he cannot sit alone and that he cannot tolerate being placed in standing, because sitting alone and tolerating being in standing are what your aims of treatment will be. Walking alone, for such a child, would be very ambitious.

Basic tone

Here you record your findings of the child's tone at rest and how it changes as he is moved or tries to move.

Postural patterns

This term is used to describe the combination of activity in different muscle groups as the child holds himself in different postures and as he moves. Under this heading you record the child's posture and movement in each of the positions in which you assessed him, and as he moved from one position to the other. For example, you might say: 'In supine, he holds his head turned mostly to the right, his shoulder girdle is retracted, his elbows are flexed and pronated (left more than right) and his hands fisted.' It is a good idea to record if, in general, the child is showing a pattern that is more flexed than extended and if one side of the body is more affected than the other.

A normal child of 1 year or more will show an endless variety of movements. Patterns of flexion and extension will be broken up and mixed together so as to be unrecognisable. It is this integration of flexion and extension that leads to the development of rotation (from 6 months onwards) that is so important for balance and coordination.

A child with spasticity, on the other hand, will show a limited variety of movements. He will use patterns that are coordinated, but not efficient or good for function because they are stereotyped or always the same. For example, if a child with spasticity tries to reach and grasp he may be able to extend his elbow, but because he moves in an abnormal stereotyped pattern this extension causes his hand to open and his forearm to pronate. He cannot, therefore, grasp an object and turn it over to look at it.

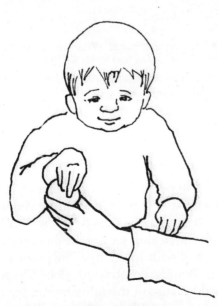

Figure 3.14
Grasping leads to flexion of the whole limb.
With normal grasp there is extension of the wrist

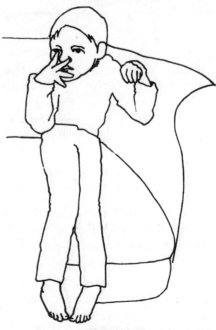

Figure 3.15
The passive extension of the knees in
this position causes the hips also to extend

The patterns that children with spasticity use to move and function are sometimes called 'total patterns'. This means that if a child starts to use an element of one pattern then the whole pattern is likely to follow. For example, if he grasps a toy with his hand this is likely to cause his whole arm to move in the flexion pattern. Again, if he is placed in long sitting his extended knees may cause his feet to plantarflex and his hips to adduct and inwardly rotate (extensor pattern), making it difficult for him to bring his trunk forward over his pelvis because the extensor pattern makes him push backwards.

The diagram below shows the mixture of patterns that can be seen in the movements of children with spasticity. For example, the upper limbs can show a flexion pattern at the same time as the lower limbs show extension; or the right side can show flexion and the left extension.

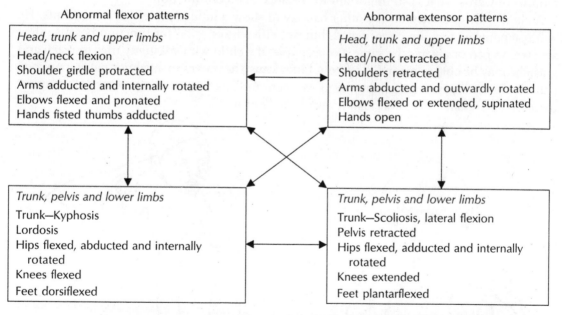

ABNORMAL PATTERNS ASSOCIATED WITH HYPERTONUS

Abnormal flexor patterns

Head, trunk and upper limbs

Head/neck flexion
Shoulder girdle protracted
Arms adducted and internally rotated
Elbows flexed and pronated
Hands fisted thumbs adducted

Trunk, pelvis and lower limbs

Trunk—Kyphosis
Lordosis
Hips flexed, abducted and internally rotated
Knees flexed
Feet dorsiflexed

Abnormal extensor patterns

Head, trunk and upper limbs

Head/neck retracted
Shoulders retracted
Arms abducted and outwardly rotated
Elbows flexed or extended, supinated
Hands open

Trunk, pelvis and lower limbs

Trunk—Scoliosis, lateral flexion
Pelvis retracted
Hips flexed, adducted and internally rotated
Knees extended
Feet plantarflexed

You may see a child using the flexion pattern in his upper limbs in combination with extension in his lower limbs. For example, in a child with spasticity in long sitting you will see that his legs are in the extension pattern, but his head may be flexed, and so too his arms and upper trunk. You may also see a child using the flexion pattern in one position and the extension pattern in another. For example, a child with spasticity lying prone may show a pattern of flexion—he is unable to lift it up, his shoulders protracted, elbows flexed, hips abducted and outwardly rotated and knees flexed because of the influence of gravity. The same child when held in standing may go up on his toes, adduct and internally rotate his hips and extend his knees (extension pattern).

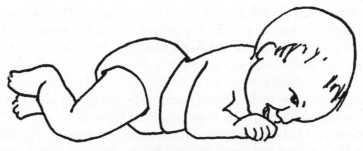

Figure 3.16
Gravity pulls child into total flexion pattern

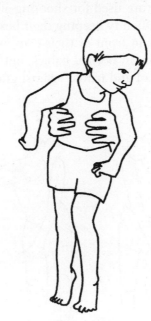

Figure 3.17
Legs are in extension pattern while arms are in flexion

These changes have causes. Very often a child with spasticity will be flexed in prone and extended in supine because of the influence of gravity. This reaction is present in a normal baby in his early weeks. It makes him flex more when the anterior surface of his body is stimulated by contact with the supporting surface, and extend more when he is on his back and it is the posterior surface of his body that is being stimulated. Normal babies lose this reaction as they become more able to come up against gravity. Children with more moderate spasticity lose it to some extent, though they may always remain under its influence. Children with severe spasticity may never be able to be free of it.

In most children with CP, the position of the head in space and in relation to the rest of the body is the other factor that can predictably influence which pattern of spasticity is seen in a child. If a child is moving only in abnormal patterns, any movement of the head will have an effect in the rest of the body. For example, a child who sits on the floor with a good deal of flexion may be in danger, when he lifts his head, of shooting over backwards. A child who can only weight-bear on his legs in standing by going into total extension may be in danger of collapsing into flexion if he flexes his head forward.

Another reaction related to head movement often occurs in children with CP. This is seen when a child's head is retracted and turned to face in one direction and the arm and leg on the opposite side flex, and on the same side extend. It is sometimes called the 'bow and arrow' posture because it is the posture used for shooting an arrow from a bow. Children who have this reaction have great difficulty keeping their heads in mid-line. They also find it hard to bring two hands together in front of their eyes or bear weight on two straight arms. This reaction is sometimes seen in normal babies, but disappears when they start to develop better extension in their head and trunk, against gravity.

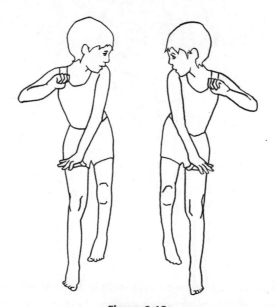

Figure 3.18
Head turning to left causes flexion pattern in right arm;
flexion pattern in left arm is caused by head turning to right

In your recording, the important thing is for you to get a clear picture of the patterns the child is using most, either to hold himself up against gravity or to move and function. In particular you will want to know which patterns he is using at home every day, when he is placed in different positions or when he moves about.

As you record the child's postural patterns, it is also important to record any asymmetry. A child who is able to use one part of his body better than others is in danger of ASSOCIATED REACTIONS. This means that the more effort he puts into using the part of his body that functions better, the greater the spasticity becomes on the more affected side. Associated reactions can also be seen when a child uses his arms to compensate for lack of movement in his legs, and the spasticity in his legs increases as a result. A child with spastic diplegia who uses a lot of effort using his arms to walk with crutches will have increased spasticity in his legs. Also, a child with hemiplegia who uses the unaffected side to function, and neglects the affected side, will have more spasticity as a result of associated reactions.

You may have noticed that children who can move about on the floor, or who can walk a little, do so in an abnormal way. Children with spasticity in their legs find it difficult to take steps and, very often, if they are crawling, find it quicker to move both legs forward at the same time. This is called bunny hopping because it is the way rabbits hop. Children who learn to walk obviously must be able to take steps, but you will have noticed that these steps are small, and the movement abnormal.

Both these ways of moving are caused by lack of DISSOCIATION between the legs. This is a result of the child using total patterns of movement. If one leg flexes, the other tends also to flex. If one leg extends so also does the other. The child who learns to walk despite these difficulties (usually a diplegic or a moderate quadriplegic) has to use a great deal of compensation by moving his trunk to make up for the lack of movement in his legs.

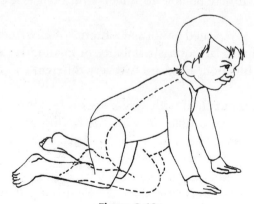

Figure 3.19
Total pattern of flexion in legs leads to lack of dissociation and bunny hopping

Contractures and deformities

A contracture is a tightening in muscles or joints that cannot be stretched without surgery. It is caused by one group of muscles pulling more powerfully than its antagonist group, over a long period of time. That is to say, it is the overuse of one abnormal pattern.

When you first see a child you will need to check all his joints and the muscles likely to be contracted, to see if he has already developed contractures. It is also, however, important to know how to anticipate which muscles and joints are likely to develop contractures.

A deformity is an abnormal position of part of the body. It involves bones, joints or soft tissue. It can be fixed or unfixed. That is, it can either be corrected passively or it cannot. You will need to note any fixed or unfixed deformities you find in the child you are assessing. There will be more information about contractures and deformities in chapter 4.

SECTION THREE

Main underlying problems

The main underlying problems relate to why a child is unable to achieve basic motor functions. As you picture the child you are assessing, you will need to identify two or three functional activities that at present he cannot do but which you think it might be possible for him to achieve with help. It is particularly important to take into account what he himself would like to be able to do and what his family would like him to be able to do. Now, looking back at your report describing his tone, patterns of movement and attitude to learning new activities, you may be able to understand the causes of his difficulties with motor function.

You may find a picture of repeated abnormal patterns of movement that is at the root of the problem, or you may find a lack of basic stability, or involuntary movements, interfering with the child's ability to function. Here are two very different examples:

- The mother of a 2-year-old child with severe spastic quadriplegia who is very irritable and who doesn't make eye contact or smile, is having great difficulty handling her child for daily care activities because he pushes back into extension with any kind of stimulation. The therapist, in her assessment, found that the child in supine turned his head always to one side and pushed vigorously back into extension with his shoulders retracted and abducted and his elbows flexed (extension pattern). His legs were somewhat flexed and abducted (PRIMITIVE). In prone, however, he could not lift his head, which was turned to one side, his back was rounded, his shoulders protracted and flexed and his hips also flexed (flexion pattern). Held in sitting he was mostly flexed, until he tried to lift his head, at which point his whole body pushed back into extension.

  In her report, under the heading of 'Main Problems', the therapist wrote that the child's spasticity was such that he could only move in total patterns that were abnormal. These patterns depended on his position, and any movement or stimulus during handling, and the position of his head, influenced the rest of his body. He could only move in response to these abnormal reactions and, therefore, could not function in a normal way.

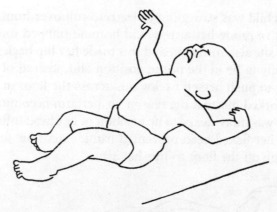

Figure 3.20
In supine: Head, shoulder girdle and arms extended, legs like newborn

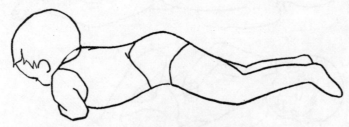

Figure 3.21
In prone: Flexion pattern

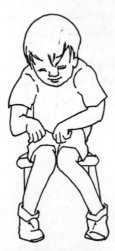

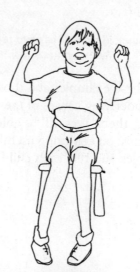

Figure 3.22
In sitting, with head flexed and arms in flexion pattern

Figure 3.23
In sitting, with head raised and arms in extension pattern

A young athetoid child was struggling to learn to roll over from supine to prone, but every time she got to prone her arm would become trapped underneath her body. If she lifted her head she also turned it, and this made her flip back into supine. This was making her unhappy to be in the prone position and, instead of learning to roll over, she was beginning to push herself backwards across the floor in supine.

The therapist worked out that the reason for her arm becoming stuck was because, in prone, her head was more flexed. The position of her head influenced the rest of her body. In this case, her flexed head prevented trunk extension, and didn't allow her to lift her body enough off the floor to free her arm.

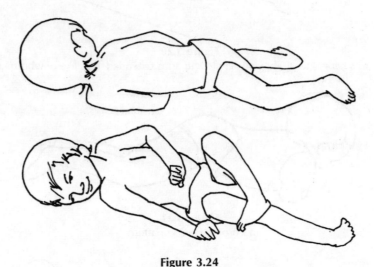

Figure 3.24
Athetoid girl rolls half into prone. Her arm gets stuck under her body and, as she lifts her head to try to free it, her head turns and she flips back into supine

I hope these examples and those in the following table will help you to understand the possible underlying causes of the problems that children with CP have. By analysing them and naming them, you will be able to better focus your efforts, as well as those of the child and his family, on achieving useful function. It is important to realise, though, that these are just examples and that each child is different.

Some possible main problems interfering with a child's motor function

Inability	Possible causes				
	In athetoid	In moderate spastic	In severe spastic	In ataxic	In child with low tone
To maintain head and trunk erect when placed in sitting or standing	• ATNR— Asymmetry • Lack of co-contraction • Involuntary movements • Poor proximal fixation • Fluctuating tone, especially with effort	• Competition of patterns (abnormal pattern of flexion combined with abnormal pattern of extension)	• Predominating pattern of flexion • Predominating pattern of extension	• Lack of sustained co-contraction • Poor proximal fixation • Unreliable balance reactions	• Poor co-contraction • Tone too low to lift trunk and head up against gravity • Pulled into gravity
To bring hands together in supine	• Asymmetrical position • Poor co-contraction preventing holding of position • Involuntary movements	• Asymmetry • Extension pattern predominating due to influence of gravity	• Extensor pattern predominating due to influence of gravity	• Poor proximal fixation • Lack of sustained co-contraction	• Insufficient tone to lift arms forward against gravity • Poor proximal fixation • Lack of sustained co-contraction
To tolerate lying prone when placed	• Active extension against gravity is not good enough to lift head • Intermittent flexor spasms may cause discomfort	• Flexion pattern likely to predominate • Intermittent flexor spasms may cause discomfort	• Gravity increases flexor spasticity and prevents active extension • Fear of not being able to lift head increases spasticity	• Poor proximal fixation • Lack of active extension leading to fear or frustration and dislike of position	• Inadequate active extension against gravity • Fear and dislike of position

(continued)

(continued)

Inability	Possible causes				
	In athetoid	In moderate spastic	In severe spastic	In ataxic	In child with low tone
To balance in sitting when placed	• Involuntary movements • Poor proximal fixation • Lack of co-contraction of head and trunk • No support of arms	• Predominance of flexion or extension • Unable to break up abnormal patterns	• Exaggerated co-contraction	• Lack of sustained co-contraction • Poor proximal fixation • Inadequate balance reactions	• Tone too low to hold body up against gravity • Poor co-contraction
To come to sitting from supine	• Inadequate flexion of head and trunk against gravity • Poor proximal fixation • Difficulty in bearing weight on arm	• Unable to break up patterns—with head flexed can't extend arm and take weight on it	• Exaggerated co-contraction	• Poor proximal fixation • Tendency to use total patterns—therefore no rotation • Poor co-contraction and difficulty in mobile weight-bearing on extended arm	• Lack of flexion against gravity • Poor co-contraction and difficulty in mobile weight-bearing on extended arm
To take steps in crawling or in standing	• Lack of co-contraction • Poor grading of movement • Poor proximal fixation • No balance • No rotation	• Use of total patterns, leading to poor dissociation between legs • No rotation	• Exaggerated co-contraction • Use of total patterns • No rotation	• Poor balance reactions • Poor proximal fixation • Poor grading of movement • No rotation	• Poor co-contraction • Lack of extension against gravity • No rotation

Chapter 4

Contractures and deformities

CONTRACTURES and deformities are major problems in treating children with cerebral palsy. It is important to understand that, except in a very few instances, the children are not born with them. They arise over time as secondary problems and, of course, they are more likely to arise where the children have less access to treatment and where referrals are late.

- A *contracture* is a permanent shortening of a muscle, muscle tendon or joint structure. A contracture becomes established once the soft tissues lose their elasticity. These peripheral tissues become increasingly fibrous, until they can only be lengthened by surgery.

- A *deformity* is an abnormal body posture or limb position. The normal alignment of one bone with another is lost and distorted, and because the child's bones are still developing, the bones themselves can grow into the distorted alignment, permanently fixing the deformity.

A growing child who cannot hold normal postures or move in normal ways is in great danger of developing contractures and deformities. This can happen very quickly if the child has spasticity and can move in only a few abnormal ways that emphasise asymmetry. But all children with CP are at risk of contractures and deformities.

As therapists, it is one of our main responsibilities to anticipate which contractures and deformities a child is in danger of developing, and then to do everything possible to prevent them. There is only a short period in a child's life in which this can be done. If we fail, the child will, sooner or later, lose functional skills already learnt. He may fail to ever learn such skills and miss the opportunity of being able to do things independently. The more severely affected children will definitely become more difficult to look after. Besides this, as the child with contractures and deformities grows into adulthood, he may be in pain because his joints are out of alignment or even dislocated, and there may also be the distress of a disfigured appearance. All in all, it is worthwhile to work hard to prevent these secondary effects of CP.

ASSESSMENT OF THREATENED OR ESTABLISHED CONTRACTURES

Principles

- *Assess the quality of the child's tone and anticipate how this will put him in danger.* Low tone can lead to deformities, because the child may be left in positions that he can't move from, or because the low tone makes his joints HYPERMOBILE and unstable.

   High tone causes abnormal patterns of movement which, if used for everyday activities and particularly if strong effort is needed, will lead to contractures and deformities.

   A child with spasticity, for example, who can move around, is likely to do so in a limited way, repeatedly using the same muscle groups and probably not moving particular joints through their full range. On the other hand, a child who is constantly moving, even if this movement is not functional or is involuntary, as in athetosis, may be less at risk of developing contractures.

- *If there is spasticity, try to extend the limited range of movement, during weight-bearing and with the child's active participation.* Once you have assessed what happens when the child moves or tries to move, you need to feel how easy or difficult it is to reach full range across the limb and across each joint in the limb. In other words, can this preferred pattern of movement of the limb be changed, and how easily? Remember that muscles often act over more than one joint.

- *Identify those positions and everyday activities that might put the child in danger.* The first step is to determine how the child usually prefers to move, where he is usually positioned during the day, how he adapts to the positions he is placed in, and how he responds to being handled (see chapter 2). The more asymmetry you observe, especially in weight-bearing, the more at risk for contractures the child is. The more effort the child uses, the tighter his muscles will be.

- *Make records so that you can monitor the danger as the child grows.*

The following example shows how to assess the extent to which a young child with right-sided hemiplegia can increase his range of movement actively, but with help.

The child might be just beginning to walk while holding on, but mostly preferring to shuffle around on his bottom. He probably *always* takes weight on the unaffected left side. He uses his unaffected left arm to prop himself and holds his right arm stiffly bent at the elbow. His right leg is turned inward at the hip. He remains like this when sitting and playing. When he walks, the same pattern repeats itself: his weight is on his left leg, his right leg is turned in at the hip, his right heel is raised and does not take weight and his right arm is stiffly bent upwards.

How easily can you help the child to change this habitual pattern? Here are some examples of how you might try:

- If he is sitting on the floor and you bend his legs a little, bringing them over to the right and keeping them there, can he adjust to this and does his right arm come down to prop himself up? If not, can you help him to do this? In this case, you are assessing whether he can accept his right hip being held in outward rotation, and how much pressure is needed to keep it there. You are also assessing his ability to overcome the preferred flexion of his right elbow and his acceptance of his right arm being extended and taking weight.

- If he is standing at a table so that he is supported and feels safe, will he reach for a toy over toward the right? Will he shift his weight on to his right leg, and keep his heel down, with your help? Will his right arm come down? Can he reach out with his right arm, overcoming the flexion?

This same way of assessing the extent of increase in range of movement can be used for all those children with spasticity who use habitual abnormal patterns for moving and playing.

You may find that you can increase the range of movement to some extent, but not to completion. Now you need to put the child you are assessing in a relaxed and comfortable position, so that you can carefully feel whether you can gain full range over the whole limb, and also feel how stiff each joint is. Perhaps his mother can read him a story or talk to him while you are doing this so that he is not anxious. As you move his limbs to feel the limitations in the muscles and soft tissues, make sure you support them in a comfortable way and keep your hands in fairly firm contact with his skin. When there is spasticity and you feel resistance, maintain your pressure until the spasticity gives a little. At the same time be careful not to fight against the spasticity and cause the child fear and pain, as this will make him tighten and will not give you a true picture of the joint limitation.

To go back to the example of the child with right hemiplegia: because of his preferred pattern of adduction and inward rotation at the hip and reluctance to take weight on the right, he is likely to have limited abduction, outward rotation and extension of his hip. Added to this, his pelvis may be retracted on the right side and he may hold it stiffly in this position even when he is lying supine. You will be able to feel this stiffness in his pelvis by bending his knees up a little and moving his pelvis in all directions (protraction, retraction, flexion, extension and side-bending). You may notice that just by moving his pelvis like this it becomes looser. If you then lift him up into standing and help him to shift the weight onto his right leg, you may find that you can get better alignment of his hip, knee and ankle and that he can now tolerate keeping his heel on the ground for a short time. Give him a lot of support so that he is not frightened but stays relaxed.

Now to assess how his abnormal pattern may have affected the length of the muscles that work on his hip and knee joints. Make him comfortable in supine and make sure that his pelvis is level. Try abducting and outwardly rotating his legs, first with his knees bent and then with them straight. Make a careful record of the range of abduction and outward rotation you can get for each leg.

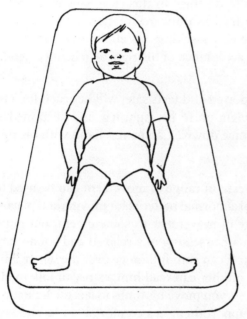 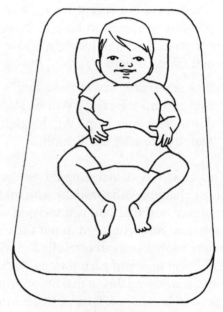

Figure 4.1
Normal limit of abduction and
outward rotation with knees straight

Figure 4.2
Normal limit of abduction and
outward rotation with knees bent

To assess him for HAMSTRING contractures, have him lie on his side with his lower leg semi-flexed at the hip and knee (Figure 4.3). This should keep his pelvis from moving. The action of the hamstrings is to extend the hip and flex the knee, so if they have become short it will be difficult to extend the knee with the hip flexed. Record how much flexion you can get at the hip with the knee straight when you move the child's upper leg.

In this position also, you can assess the length of the child's hip flexors. With the pelvis fixed it should be possible to bring the child's upper leg to 15 degrees of extension beyond the midline. Make sure that the leg is neither adducted nor abducted, and in neutral rotation.

You already checked the lengthening ability of the CALF MUSCLES and ACHILLES TENDON when you helped the child to shift weight onto his right leg in standing with his heel down. Perhaps it was difficult to get his heel to come down completely, or perhaps he compensated for his inability to do this by flexing his hip and knee. Now feel how much resistance there

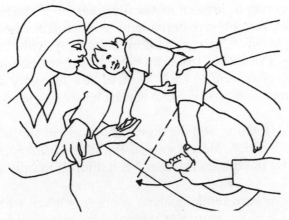

Figure 4.3
Assessing the length of the hamstrings

is when you stretch his calf muscles and Achilles tendon while he lies in supine. Remember that the calf muscles flex the knee and plantarflex the ankle, so you must have the knee in extension while you dorsiflex the ankle, pulling the calcaneus downwards so that you stretch the Achilles tendon and not the structures of the foot.

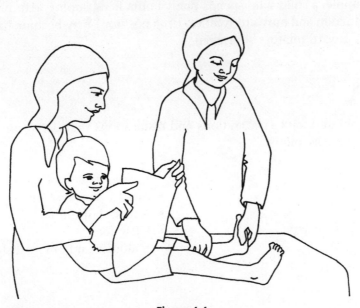

Figure 4.4
Feeling the limitations of stretch in the calf muscle and Achilles tendon

The same principles may be applied to assessing present or threatening contractures in the child's upper limbs. First observe his patterns of movement when he tries to reach out and grasp an object, or when he tries to prop himself up with one arm while he uses his other hand to play. Can you increase this range by helping him to shift weight or keep his arm extended as he takes weight on it? Does it make a difference if you first mobilise his shoulder girdle and upper DORSAL SPINE? Can you get his SCAPULA to move, or does he hold it very stiffly?

Later, with the child in sitting, feel the degree of stiffness in all the joints and muscles as you elevate and abduct the shoulder. Can you get full outward rotation with the arm in SUPINATION and the wrist and fingers extended? Is it difficult to fully abduct and OPPOSE THE THUMB?

So far we have mostly been thinking about younger children with moderate spasticity. With these children, we have a particular responsibility to anticipate contractures as they learn to move and function with their own kind of coordination. In the case of older children who have not been able to get treatment, and in the case of younger children with severe spasticity, our objective must be to record the extent of the contractures we see and prevent them from getting worse (see chapter 5).

Children with very low tone can also develop contractures, but these will be slow to develop and can be anticipated by observing the positions in which the child is habitually placed. For example, a child who spends many hours lying supine with his legs pulled by gravity into abduction and outward rotation (frog position) may become fixed, and his hip abductors and outward rotators shortened.

DEFORMITIES

The bony changes and joint subluxations and dislocations that occur most frequently in children with CP are as follows:

- Scoliosis
- Kyphosis
- Lordosis
- Subluxation of the hip
- Hip dislocation

- HYPEREXTENSION of the knee
- PATELLA displacement
- Rocker bottom feet
- Claw toes
- Shoulder and elbow dislocation

Scoliosis

A scoliosis is a deformity of the spine that causes a sideways curve. It occurs when the muscles of the trunk pull down more on one side than the other. The children who are found to have the worst scolioses are those with fluctuating tone. A child with fluctuating tone usually has great difficulty holding her trunk and head erect. So, for safety, her mother is likely to leave her lying in supine on the floor. In this position the child may learn to roll onto her side, but she is likely to be able to roll more easily to one side than the other. In time, the pull down in the favoured side of her trunk will cause a fixed scoliosis.

Once a child has a fixed scoliosis it is even more difficult for her to actively extend her trunk. It is also very difficult to place her in a good sitting position. Meanwhile, the scoliosis becomes more and more pronounced until the child's breathing becomes restricted and she becomes prone to chest infections.

Less severe scolioses are seen in children with hemiplegia, diplegia or moderate quadriplegia. In these cases, the scoliosis will be caused by the imbalance of muscle pull in the trunk, or by the shortening of one leg caused by the child's not taking weight as much on that side as on the other. All scolioses, including the less severe, will lead to back pain and loss of movement of the spine later in life.

Kyphosis

Kyphosis describes a forward curve of the upper spine into flexion. A child may develop it to compensate for a lordosis, or he may develop a kyphosis as a result of flexor spasticity of the trunk. A child with spasticity who is placed in prone will try to lift his head, but because the flexion pattern always predominates in prone and because of the effect of using effort, his flexor spasticity will increase. This will make it very difficult for him to actively extend his head and trunk.

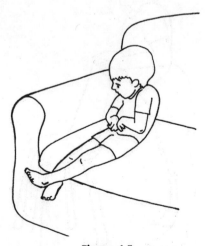

Figure 4.5
Flexion in upper limbs and trunk to compensate for too much extension in lower limbs causes kyphosis in a child with spastic quadriplegia

Children who can't sit up alone are often propped up, in sitting, in the corner of a chair or sofa. If they are placed with a straight trunk and hips flexed at right angles it is most likely that they will flop forwards or be pulled forward by flexor spasticity, and may even fall on to the floor. For this reason, most mothers leave their children with their hips in some extension and their trunks leaning backwards, supported by a cushion. But if from this position the child tries to move forwards to reach with his hands, he will only be able to flex from his upper trunk and shoulders. This is because of the mainly extensor pattern in his legs. He may be able to use his hands a little in this way, but all the time the spasticity will be increasing in his trunk, putting him in danger of a fixed kyphosis.

Lordosis

Lordosis is overextension of the spine in the lumbar region so that the back is hollowed at waist level. A child who cannot actively extend her hips when placed in standing is likely to hyperextend her knees and extend her lumbar spine to compensate. This is frequently found in a child with diplegia whose trunk is inactive and whose pelvis has become fixed and immobile. The lordosis can become fixed if the child has to use this pattern to walk about a lot.

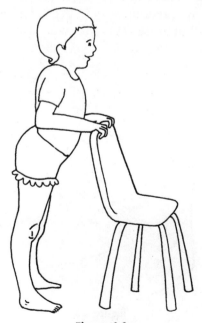

Figure 4.6
Lordosis develops either in compensation for kyphosis or as a means of
bringing the trunk upright when active hip extension is not adequate

Subluxation of the hip

Subluxation happens in a joint when one bone slips in and out of place.

In all new-born babies, the ACETABULUM is shallow and insubstantial. It becomes properly able to hold the head of the FEMUR only if the baby moves his legs against the pelvis in kicking and later takes weight on his legs either in crawling or standing. It is the movement of the weighted head of the femur that deepens and shapes the bony cup that will hold it in place. A child who does not have the opportunity to stand and move may therefore be in danger of having an inadequately formed acetabulum, and the head of his femur may slip in and out. When he is young this may not cause any problems or discomfort, but he is sure to experience pain as he gets older, especially if the head of the femur is pulled out of its place by spasms.

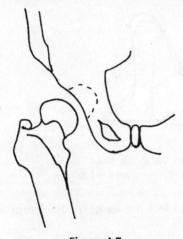

Figure 4.7
In a normal baby, during the first year the head of the femur deepens the cup of the acetabulum

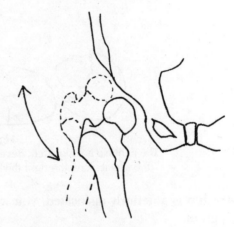

Figure 4.8
Without full range of abduction and outward rotation, the acetabulum is shallow and the femur is not held in place

The best way to assess the stability of a child's hip joint is to have it X-rayed. If the head of the femur is shown in the X-ray to be almost all covered by the acetabulum, the joint is stable. The more uncovered it is, the more unstable it is.

Hip dislocation

This is more serious than subluxation. When the hip is dislocated, the head of the femur stays outside the acetabulum. It may be displaced either ANTERIORLY or POSTERIORLY. If it is anteriorly dislocated, it sits below and medial to the anterior superior iliac spine. If it is posteriorly dislocated, it sits above and behind the acetabulum. Posterior dislocation is more common and is mostly seen in children who flex, adduct and inwardly rotate their hips with spasticity in order to function. A child who is in danger of this will be one who rarely takes weight on her legs and who lies in supine with WINDSWEPT hips. The hip that is more adducted and inwardly rotated is in most danger. Anterior dislocation is mostly seen in children who spend a good deal of their time lying supine with their legs in a frog position (hips abducted, flexed and outwardly rotated).

If is not possible to see an X-ray of the child's hip, it may be possible to feel when the hip is dislocated. To assess a child for a posteriorly dislocated hip, place him in supine and make sure that his pelvis is level. Flex both of his legs so that his feet are on the floor and his legs together. If he has a dislocated hip, the affected leg will appear to be much shorter, and the GREATER TROCHANTER will be more prominent on the affected side, and higher and more posterior than on the unaffected side.

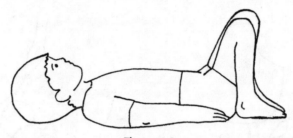

Figure 4.9
The right hip is dislocated. Because the head of the femur is outside the acetabulum, the right thigh seems much shorter than the left

If the hip is anteriorly dislocated, you will be able to feel the head of the femur in the child's groin.

A child who has a dislocated hip is very difficult to place in a normal, comfortable sitting position. This is because it is difficult for the hip to be flexed to a right angle. As the child gets older she may also suffer pain and discomfort in the hip joint.

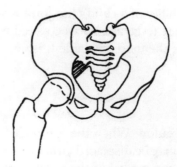

Figure 4.10
Head of femur in normal position in deep acetabulum

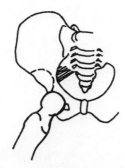

Figure 4.11
Head of femur dislocated anteriorly

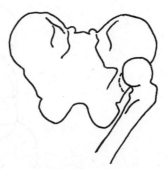

Figure 4.12
Head of femur dislocated posteriorly

Hyperextension of the knee

This happens when the structures at the back of the knee joint become lax and allow the knee to overextend. It is often seen in a child with low tone who compensates for inadequate hip extension by locking her knees in extension (Figure 4.13).

However, it can also be seen in a child with a tight Achilles tendon who can only get her heel to the ground, while walking, by hyperextending the knee. Another but rather less common reason for hyperextension of the knee is if the hamstring tendons have been over-released during surgery.

Patella displacement

The patella (kneecap) is a small bone enclosed in the lower end of the QUADRICEPS MUSCLE. If there is an unequal pull on either the medial or the lateral head of the quadriceps, the patella will be displaced and will not be able to function as an efficient lever for straightening the knee.

Children who are able to walk alone, but who walk with slightly flexed knees (crouch gait), very often develop pain in their knees (Figure 4.14). This is caused by the patella being drawn upwards and away from its usual position in relation to the femur. It can even result in the child being unable to continue walking .

Rocker bottom feet

This deformity gives the child's foot the appearance of the rocker bottom of a rocking chair. It is caused by the child's difficulty in getting his heel to the ground because he is using the abnormal pattern of extension (which includes plantarflexion at his ankle) to hold himself

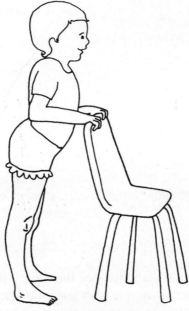

Figure 4.13
This child has poor active hip extension. She compensates with
hyperextension of her knees and lordosis (hollowing of the back)

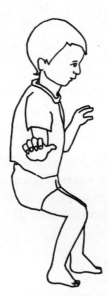

Figure 4.14
Crouch gait describes the way a child walks when his knees and hips are always slightly bent

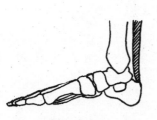

Figure 4.15
Bony arch of a normal foot

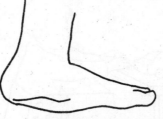

Figure 4.16
Rocker bottom foot deformity

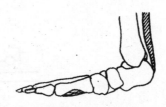

Figure 4.17
Bone position in rocker bottom foot

up against gravity. The arch of his foot flattens to compensate. Over time, the weight of his body habitually pressing down on the arch reverses its curve. By the time he reaches adulthood, the changes in the joints and ligaments of his feet will cause him pain.

To prevent rocker bottom feet, you must first reduce the spasticity in his hips and pelvis and give him better active extension against gravity. Some weight-bearing every day with his feet and legs in a good position and the possibility of active extension in his hips will help. You must teach him how to stretch his own Achilles tendon in weight-bearing. In general, you also need to make sure that all children who cannot actively lift up the long arch of their feet are given shoes with arch supports.

Claw toes

Toes that are held in flexion can become fixed in a kind of claw position. This is either because of predominantly flexor spasticity or to compensate for poor coordination of the leg and trunk muscles in the child's efforts to balance. Eventually it will not be possible to fully straighten out the toes, and this will mean the child will have a less stable base for standing. The bent toes may also be difficult to fit into shoes.

If you notice a child standing with his toes held mostly in flexion, you can prevent claw toes becoming a fixed deformity by placing a small lift under his toes inside his shoes, and by using felt or sponge to hold his toes in abduction.

Shoulder and elbow dislocation

These are most likely to occur in children with low or fluctuating tone, especially those children whose dystonic spasms throw them into extreme postures.

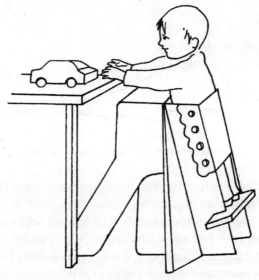

Figure 4.18
Spending time in a forward-leaning standing frame with arch supports or ankle foot orthoses
prevents rocker bottom foot deformity and encourages active extension of hips and knees

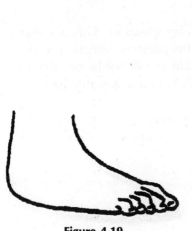

Figure 4.19
Claw toes

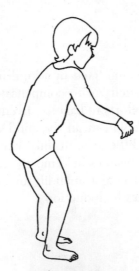

Figure 4.20
This girl is flexing her toes to
compensate for poor control
of hips and knees

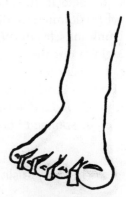

Figure 4.21
Separating toes with sponge
wedges may prevent claw toes

SOME ASSISTIVE DEVICES THAT CAN BE USED TO PREVENT CONTRACTURES AND DEFORMITIES

Splints

This book cannot cover this subject in much depth. Where there are resources and good orthotic expertise, there will be a wide choice of splinting available, especially for children who walk up on their toes. Where there is some orthotic expertise and where light plastic material is available, it is worthwhile making ankle foot ORTHOSES (AFOs) for these children. The aim is for the AFO to hold the heel in alignment (not allowing it to swing MEDIALLY or LATERALLY) and to prevent plantarflexion of the foot during walking. The child wears the AFO inside her boot or shoe, and she will need a larger size than normal to accommodate it. It must be a very good fit and it is the therapist's responsibility to see that it does not cause pressure sores.

It is important to remember that if the AFO holds the foot in DORSIFLEXION, this is likely to increase the child's tendency to also flex the hip and knee. Therefore, while wearing AFOs, a child must be encouraged to actively extend hips and knees.

It has recently been noted that using AFOs for long periods every day can cause wasting of the calf muscles, so a balance should be found between correcting the ankle position and keeping the calf muscles exercised.

Footwear

Medical boots are often heavy and may look unattractive. If they are not achieving a useful purpose for a child, try to avoid them. A child whose ankle joint INVERTS or EVERTS when weight-bearing may be helped by a well-fitting boot. If a boot has a narrow-enough heel that grips the CALCANEOUS, this can also help to prevent plantarflexion; but not many boots will fit the child in this way. Well-fitting shoes with an arch support are probably the most advisable footwear for the majority of children. They should wear these as soon as they start spending any part of the day in standing.

When putting on shoes, have the child in sitting on a stool with his knee flexed to a right angle and his foot on the floor. Make sure the shoe is wide open. If you can, slip your finger under his toes to make sure they are not flexed. If this is impossible, push down on the child's knee while feeling through the shoe to see if his toes are flexed. When you are sure the toes are straight, fasten the shoe.

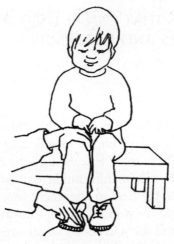

Figure 4.22
Pressure on the knee down through the leg will reduce the spasticity in the toes.
Fasten the shoe only when you are sure the toes are straight

Callipers

In places where it is difficult to make light plastic orthoses, doctors sometimes prescribe long leg CALLIPERS for children who cannot stand alone. While this may be helpful in holding the child's knees in extension and their heels on the ground, it is likely to increase the spasticity around the hips and pelvis. If the child then tries to walk while wearing the callipers it will be very difficult and the effort will further increase the spasticity. Where callipers might be useful would be to hold the child's legs in extension while she stands in a standing frame or at a table. But callipers are expensive to make, and the cost in such a case may not be justified.

CAN SURGERY HELP TO CORRECT CONTRACTURES AND DEFORMITIES?

Surgery should only be done if all other efforts fail in elongating tight muscles. It is better to do surgery when the child is more then 8 years old so that it will not need to be done again as she grows.

It is important to remember that contractures and deformities are caused by the everyday postures and movement the child prefers. Even if tendons and the right muscles are elongated surgically, the problem will recur unless you help the child to move in a more normal way.

All surgery does damage and leaves muscles weaker than before. But this is preferable to the pain caused by sub-luxated or dislocated joints. If there is X-ray evidence that the head of the femur is less and less covered by the acetabulum, release of the adductor muscles and ilio-psoas can reduce the risk of dislocation. Subluxation or dislocation is not likely in children who walk alone. It is more likely in children who walk with aids, and most likely in those who don't walk at all. Children with spastic quadriplegia who sit with windswept hips are in danger of having one hip dislocate posteriorly and the other anteriorly.

If the Achilles tendons need lengthening this should not be done before the child is 8 years old. After surgery the plaster cast should hold the ankle at 0-degree, and not 5-degree or 10-degree dorsiflexion. The child should not wear the cast for more than 2–4 weeks. She should walk as soon as the cast is dry.

In all cases of surgery for children with CP, there must be good communication between surgeon, therapist and family, so that the reasons for surgery are well understood by the family and the therapist can follow the surgeon's plan for the child responsibly.

Chapter 5

Principles of treatment

THE most important thing to know and understand about treating children with CP is that each child needs his own programme and no one child is the same as another. It is not possible to say, 'This child has diplegia, therefore this set of exercises is what he needs.' This is because one child with diplegia will function in a different way to any other. Also, the way to make changes to one child's abnormal tone and postural patterns, to meet his needs and deal with his problems, may be different to the way that works with another child. The same is true for all the different kinds of CP. That is what makes treating these children such a challenge.

In order to meet this challenge, we are going to consider the principles governing the range of treatment techniques that we can use to increase and improve the child's functional abilities and prevent contractures and deformities. In the next chapter, we will look at how treatment can be adapted to fit the circumstances that the child and his family find themselves in.

Before you can do that, though, you have to know what treatment may be effective and how you can carry it out. In order to be effective, your treatment programme should:

- *Prepare the child for function at her appropriate level.*
  By 'level', I mean what is appropriate for her developmental stage and her needs. Treatment should prepare her to achieve a specific goal that will give a better quality of life for her or her family, but that is within her developmental stage and intellect.

- *Incorporate the child's own activity into the treatment.*
  Enable her to be active either in holding a position or moving. Help her to start an interesting or challenging activity, then gradually withdraw support so she carries on alone.

- *Make tone more normal to make coordination possible.*
  By handling and guiding the activities of the child, we can reduce the spasticity in a child with raised tone, increase tone in a child who is hypotonic, and make the tone more steady in a child who is athetoid or ataxic.

- *Give the child sensory experience of more normal movement.*
  Helping the child to move and play with better coordination will give him the feeling of what is normal. The more often he can carry out that more normal movement, the

more it will be laid down in his central nervous system and the easier it will become for him.

HOW DO WE MAKE TONE MORE NORMAL?

When a child has spasticity or athetosis, he moves in abnormal patterns which may not be functional. We can enable the child to function better while counteracting any unwanted increase in tone by the use of positioning, weight-bearing, handling and movement.

Positioning a child with CP in supine, as we have seen in our assessment, increases extensor tone. In prone, the FLEXOR TONE is increased. We can use this knowledge in treatment. For example, we would not treat a child with strong flexor spasms in prone on the floor unless we could reduce those spasms in some way. Similarly, it would be very difficult to treat a child who pushes back into extension in supine on the floor. In treatment, we position the child in ways that change the abnormal patterns. We do this by changing one, or maybe two, elements of the abnormal pattern and substituting a part of a different pattern. These altered patterns are called *tone-influencing patterns* (TIPs). Imagine a child with moderate quadriplegia placed in cross-legged sitting on the floor. His head will be pulled down, his shoulders protracted and his arms flexed and pronated. He cannot balance much, nor can he reach forward for a toy or even lift his head to look around him.

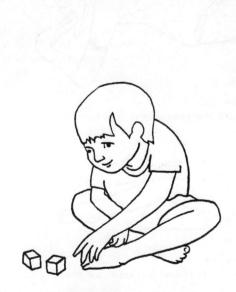

Figure 5.1
Child in cross-legged sitting. Too much flexion prevents him from reaching out with his hands

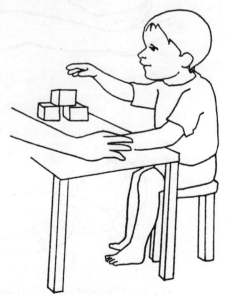

Figure 5.2
When he sits up on a chair the pattern is broken (his legs are not abducted and outwardly rotated), so he can reach better

If, however, we take away one or two elements of the flexion pattern (abduction and outward rotation of his legs) and place him in sitting on a stool, provided he can extend his trunk he will be able to balance and use his hands better. This is because his legs are now less flexed, less outwardly rotated and more adducted. The flexion pattern is altered.

Another example is a child who pushes back into extension in supine. Her head is extended and turned to one side, her legs adducted, extended and inwardly rotated, and her mother has great difficulty abducting her legs in order to change her nappy. If she flexed her head forward by placing it on a small pillow, this might be enough to change her pattern of extension, and her legs would more easily flex and abduct.

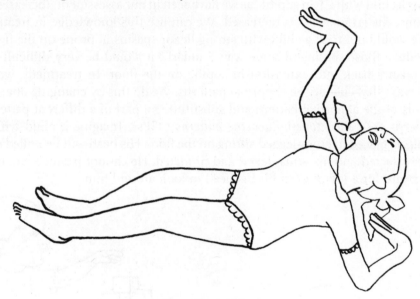

Figure 5.3
For this girl, when she lies on her back, the extension pattern takes over

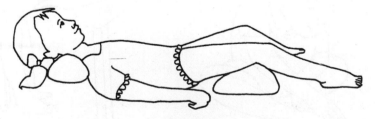

Figure 5.4
The extension pattern is changed when her head and knees are flexed

When we put a child in a position we have to also consider the subject of *mobile weight-bearing*. Positioning a child in such a way that he is helped to bear weight through his limbs or trunk, and at the same time he moves (or is moved) a little, will reduce spasticity and prepare him to maintain functional postures. For example, a child who has some flexor spasticity and finds it difficult to lift his head when placed in prone may be helped by being placed on a mobile surface, such as a roll. This position also gives him the possibility of taking some weight through his extended arms, which further reduces the pull down in his shoulders.

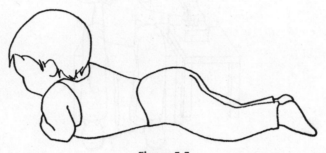

Figure 5.5
Arms flexed under body increase flexor spasticity

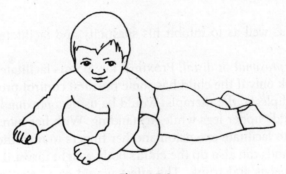

Figure 5.6
Mobile weight-bearing on arms reduces spasticity

A child with athetosis or ataxia placed in standing, and bearing weight through an extended arm on a table in front, will have more possibility of symmetry and coordinated co-contraction because the weight-bearing, as he moves and plays, regulates his tone and controls OVERSHOOTING.

We have seen that by using positions we can not only reduce a child's spasticity, we can also facilitate more normal postures and movements. The key to further facilitation is through *handling*. The way we touch and move the child will have a very powerful effect, so we must make sure that this effect is good. It helps to know that through just one point at any one time, we can control and change the child's posture and pattern of movement. These points are called *key points of control*. They are the points where we place our hands in order to

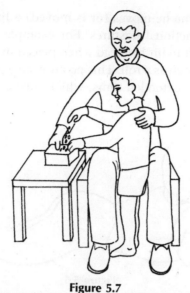

Figure 5.7
Mobile weight-bearing on legs regulates the tone of a child with athetosis

stimulate the child, as well as to inhibit his spasticity and facilitate normal postures and movements.

Key points can be *proximal* or *distal*. Proximal key points facilitate more activity distally. Distal keypoints work only if the child has some postural control proximally. In the case of a child with spastic diplegia, the therapist would be using a *proximal keypoint* if she placed her hands on the child's upper legs while in standing. With her hands in this position she can use her thumbs to facilitate extension and her fingers to turn the child's hips into outward rotation. Her hands can also tip the child's body weight forward to get good alignment in the lower limbs, pelvis and trunk. The effect would be to reduce the spasticity in the lower limbs and facilitate hip extension and weight-bearing through feet with heels flat on the floor.

An example of a *distal keypoint* would be in a child with hemiplegia, where the therapist uses the child's hand, in particular the base of the thumb on the hemiplegic side, to change the abnormal pattern of movement in the whole arm. At the same time, she can shift the child's weight over on to the hemiplegic leg. This will only be effective if the child has good enough proximal activity to allow him to accommodate to the stimulation.

Examples of proximal key points of control are the *head, spine,* STERNUM, *shoulder girdle* and *pelvis/hips.* Some distal key points are *jaw, wrists, knees, fingers, base of thumbs, ankles* and *big toes.*

But *how* do we use the key points of control? What should we do with our hands when they are placed on the chosen point?

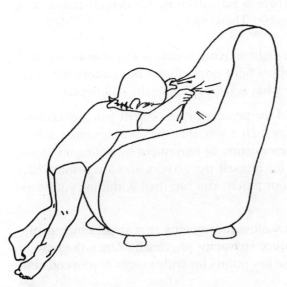

Figure 5.8
Child with diplegia uses functionally better arms to pull to stand. This increases extensor spasticity in legs

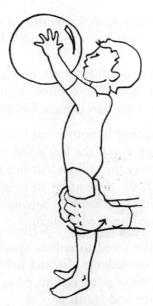

Figure 5.9
Therapist reduces spasticity, stimulates activity and facilitates extension and weight-bearing through proximal keypoint

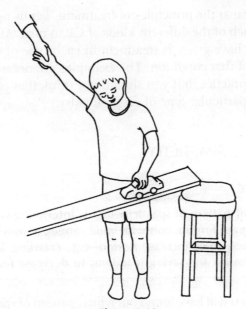

Figure 5.10
In a child with hemiplegia the therapist uses distal keypoint of control (base of thumb) to outwardly rotate, extend and supinate the arm, at the same time facilitating weight-bearing on the affected leg

It is not easy to describe this in writing. There is no substitute for demonstration and practical training but a few guidelines are possible. These are:

- Keep your hands firmly on the child. A light moving touch is too stimulating and cannot be used to control or guide. Equally, a tight grip will not be comfortable or effective. Your hands must feel all the time what is happening in the child's body.

- Keep clearly in your mind the elements of the posture or movement you are working for. Keep using the key point of control in such a way that the child becomes active. Remember the child is learning a whole new posture or movement by feeling it happen in his body. If he starts to be able to do for himself the activity you are helping him with, you will feel him become light to your touch. You can then withdraw your support until he needs it again.

- Move the child to reduce spasticity. Fairly slow movements in a small range in the trunk, shoulder girdle and pelvis will reduce spasticity proximally. Once the tone in the proximal parts is reduced you must use key points for wide ranges of movement in the limbs and trunk.

- Use your hands to support the child in positions that will be useful for him, while stimulating him to be active in other parts of his body.

We have looked in general at the principles of treatment. Let us now look at how we can apply those principles to each of the different kinds of CP in turn. At this point I must issue a warning. The examples I have given as treatment in each type of CP *must not* be seen as 'recipes' for the treatment of that condition. The examples are necessary to illustrate a way of putting a principle into practice, but you should not think that each example is the one and only way to treat that particular type of cerebral palsy.

CHILDREN WITH SEVERE SPASTICITY

Principles of treatment

- **Analyse the predominant pattern of spasticity that is interfering with function**
- **Use patterns which prepare for function with wide ranges of movement**
- **Avoid functional activities which increase flexion—e.g., crawling, kneeling, W-sitting**
- **Work for righting, EQUILIBRIUM and saving reactions, to decrease fear**

Through your assessment, you will have found out which pattern of spasticity is predominant. In the child with severe spasticity this may be flexion or extension, or the child may be almost rigid when both flexion and extension are equally present. In the predominantly *flexed* child you will see a fairly symmetrical position, although there is likely to be more side flexion in one side of the trunk than the other and the pelvis will be retracted on that side. If you remember, in children with severe spasticity the tone is higher proximally than distally, so your first objective is to reduce the tone in the trunk, pelvis and shoulder girdle and then work in the pattern which will prepare the child for function. In the case of the flexed child, the danger of contractures is great even in very young children. You must therefore use every position and situation you can think of to get the child extended. Use gravity to help you and, once you have got the child in an extended position, use keypoints to facilitate his actively extending and abducting his limbs in wide ranges of movement and bearing weight through limbs and trunk.

There is no avoiding the fact that all this takes time. But if you can find the most effective way to help the mother make her child with severe spasticity looser and easier to handle, she will agree that it is time well spent.

Possible positions in which to treat flexed child with severe spasticity

1. *Supine, head down on mother's legs* (if the child is small enough). In this position gravity facilitates extension, and if the mother moves her legs a little it will help to reduce the spasticity.

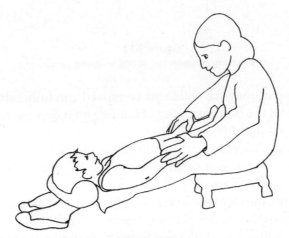

Figure 5.11
Mother moves her own legs one after the other to reduce the
spasticity in the child's trunk. Gravity facilitates extension

2. *Side lying on mother's knee on side that is more flexed.* If that side is elongated before the child is put in position, the weight-bearing will reduce the spasticity. In this position the child can be facilitated to reach out with his upper arm and to kick into extension

and abduction with his upper leg. Later, he can perhaps be helped to roll into prone and lift his head and trunk.

3. *Carrying in side-lying position.* As the child is lifted and moved from place to place at home, this way of carrying can be good treatment. The more flexed side is kept elongated and the mother's arm between the child's legs keeps them abducted, outwardly rotated and extended. Holding the child like this, but more into prone, will make it possible for him to lift his head and trunk against gravity, as long as the flexor spasticity can be reduced.

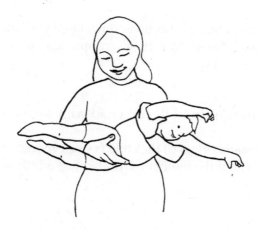

Figure 5.12
Carrying position for strongly flexed child

From these starting positions the child can be moved carefully into any other position that you feel will give him the best possibility of holding an independent posture or carrying out some activity that satisfies him.

Predominantly extended children are very difficult for mothers to handle. They push backwards with their heads, and sometimes their whole bodies, against the mother's arm when she is trying to hold or carry them.

One way is to have the mother tuck him under her arm, holding his legs in flexion, abduction and outward rotation. In this position his head will have nothing to push against, and the mother's arm around his shoulders will keep them in protraction. This, combined with holding his hips in flexion, should break up the pattern of total extension.

Feeding can be extremely difficult too because, as the child pushes back into extension, his mouth opens and his tongue pushes forwards. A good position that changes this is to have the child sitting between his mother's knees, while she sits on the floor. The child's hips and knees are a little flexed. His mother keeps his shoulders forward and also presses her hand against his sternum. This is a good key point from which to reduce neck retraction.

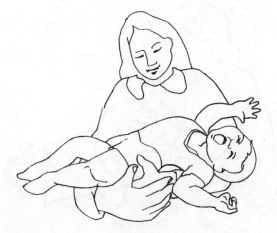

Figure 5.13
Difficulty in controlling a child with severe extensor spasticity

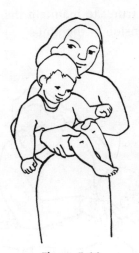

Figure 5.14
Possible alternative carrying position

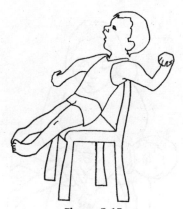

Figure 5.15
Severe extensor thrust makes
seating and feeding difficult

There is a danger, though, that children with severe spasticity who have patterns of total extension, can suddenly develop a flexion pattern instead. It is important, therefore, to begin working as soon as possible for active extension of the head and trunk against gravity, and also extension, abduction and outward rotation of the limbs. A good way to do this is to place the child in prone across your knees. Slight movement of your knees will inhibit flexor spasticity. Use the shoulder girdle or pelvis as a key point of control to rotate the trunk and make it possible for the child to lift his head, thereby getting active extension in

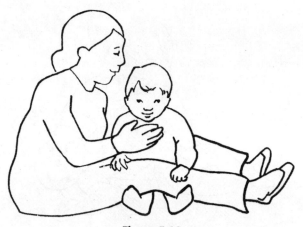

Figure 5.16
Alternative position for feeding or play

his whole trunk. You can later use your forearm on the trunk to maintain the extension, while freeing your hands to facilitate abduction and extension of the limbs.

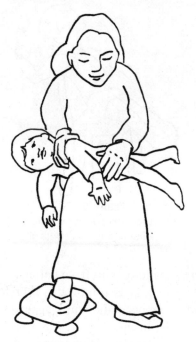

Figure 5.17
Reducing spasticity in the trunk using rotation

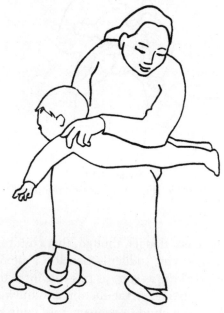

Figure 5.18
Using forearm to maintain extension, leaving hands free

Another big problem with extended children is that they are in great danger of hip dislocation because of the spastic pattern of adduction and internal rotation of their legs. This pattern also makes it difficult for the mother to change the child's nappies. These two problems can be alleviated at the same time if the mother can use the nappy-changing time to change the pattern of spasticity.

She can do this by having the child lie in supine with her head flexed forward on a small folded towel. She may also need to place something under each shoulder to protract the shoulder girdle. It should be possible to bring her hands down to her sides at least momentarily. Once she has adjusted to the position the mother can start working on her legs, but she should keep talking to her so that she learns to enjoy the position.

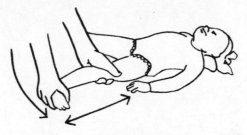

Figure 5.19
Step 1: Bring the first leg into outward rotation and abduction
and then push the whole leg upwards into the acetabulum

To begin with, the mother tips the child's pelvis forward and backward a little to mobilise it. Then she works on one leg to bring it into as much outward rotation, extension and abduction in the hip as she can with the knee in extension and, if possible, the foot in dorsiflexion. She pushes upwards through the leg to push the head of the femur into the acetabulum

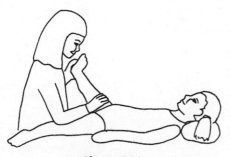

Figure 5.20
Step 2: Hold the first leg in position with
forearm while bringing the second leg into
abduction and outward rotation

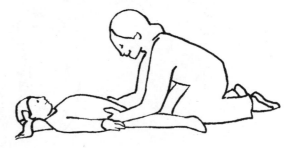

Figure 5.21
Step 3: Keeping both legs in position with
forearms, help the child to actively
lift her bottom off the floor

(Figure 5.19). This action also reduces the spasticity. She then keeps the leg in this position with her forearm while she does the same thing with the other leg (Figure 5.20). Finally, she rests both forearms on the child's thighs to hold the whole position and uses her hands to lift her pelvis. At the same time, she can ask the child to help her lift her bottom (Figure 5.21). All this will not happen in just the right way the first time it is tried. It may take weeks, but it will become easier each day.

This exercise to reduce spasticity and facilitate active extension with abduction of the hips is good preparation for placing the child in standing. The child should be lifted into a

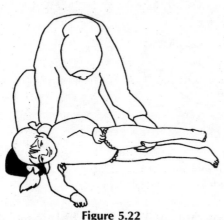

Figure 5.22
Step 1: Roll child onto her side and lift her without flexing hips or knees. Hold her close to your body

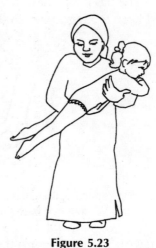

Figure 5.23
Step 2: Keep holding her in extension as you bring her into a standing position

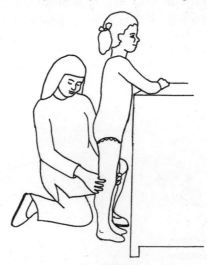

Figure 5.24
Step 3: Place her in standing, still keeping her in extension

standing without allowing any flexion to happen in the hips and knees. You will find the child can now more easily actively extend her hips and knees than if you had done no preparation.

CHILDREN WITH MODERATE SPASTICITY

Principles of treatment

- **Reduce tone by countering the patterns of spasticity and by avoiding too much stimulation and effort**
- **Avoid using stereotyped patterns of movement for function—find ways to break them up**
- **Facilitate sequences of movement**
- **Facilitate wide ranges of movement in tone-influencing patterns (TIPs)**

The main danger that children with *moderate spasticity* face is that, as they grow and become more challenged to achieve independence, they will use their abnormal patterns of movement to function and their spasticity will increase. The reason the spasticity increases is that they are using more and more effort. The more effort they use, the more *associated reactions* they will acquire. That is, the more they use the less affected parts of their bodies, the more the spasticity will increase in the more affected parts.

In a young child, we have the opportunity to prevent the worst of this effect. This is not to say that we can make the child normal, but we can prevent the escalating buildup of spasticity and the neglect of the affected parts. This, in turn, will help to prevent contractures and deformities.

Knowing how the child functions at home or at school is very important. A child with moderate spasticity who spends a good deal of his time crawling with very flexed legs will have difficulty learning to walk. Rather than crawling, this child must have a walking aid that supports him in a standing position and allows him to take some weight on his legs in the correct position and to move around independently. This will prepare him for walking, whereas crawling is more likely to prevent it.

Whatever abnormal pattern we see the child using, we must work to counteract it. This should be done not just in treatment, but much more importantly, in everyday life as well. The young child with hemiplegia who learns to bottom shuffle in side sitting, retracting his affected side behind him, must be facilitated to take weight on his affected side in sitting, standing and in sequences of movement. He must also have opportunities to take weight on his affected arm and outstretched hand while he plays. This will not only result in better function, it will also help to prevent *associated reactions* brought about by his efforts to play using just his unaffected hand.

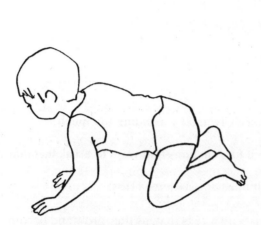

Figure 5.25
Crawling, using too much flexion

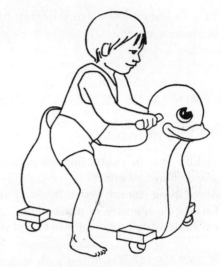

Figure 5.26
Taking weight on the feet and pushing
on the ground facilitates extension and is
a better way for the child to move around

Mobile weight-bearing is the key to a child being able to change from one position to another. Children with moderate spasticity need help to take weight on limbs with abnormally high tone. Once they can be placed with weight through the limb, however, the trunk can be moved (by the mother or therapist) against the limb (Figures 5.27 and 5.28). This not only reduces the spasticity, it is also very good sensori-motor experience for the child. This is preparation for sequences of movement.

Some children with moderate spasticity experience *flexor spasms* in their hips. These are uncomfortable, even painful, and children soon learn to be apprehensive about being placed in the positions that they know can cause them. Fear increases the possibility of spasms occurring, so it will be necessary for you to make sure that a child's treatment is at all times interesting and satisfying for him. The spasms are less likely to happen if you are able to prepare the child first by reducing the flexor spasticity at the hips. You can do this with the child in prone by pressing down on his sacrum and rocking him a little from side to side to rotate the spine. Those children who have spasms when lying prone on the floor will be easier to treat across their mother's knees or over a large roll or ball (Figures 5.29 and 5.30). This is because they will be lying on a mobile surface and the movement reduces the spasticity.

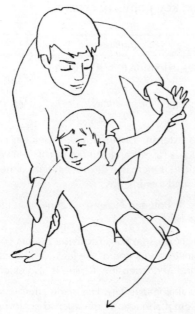

Figure 5.27
Therapist facilitates child to take weight on her right arm. He uses abduction and outward rotation of left arm to reduce spasticity, and from this point rotates the trunk against the weight-bearing arm

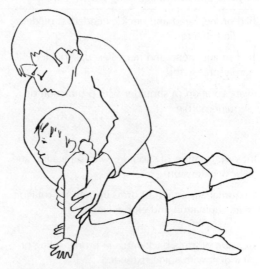

Figure 5.28
It is then quite easy to place her weight-bearing through two outstretched arms. He can later take her back to side-sitting so that she gets the experience of changing her position from side-sitting to crawling and back

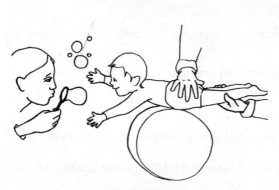

Figure 5.29
Therapist holds legs in extension, presses down on child's sacrum and moves the child slightly backwards and forwards on the roll. This reduces the flexor spasms and facilitates extension in his head and trunk

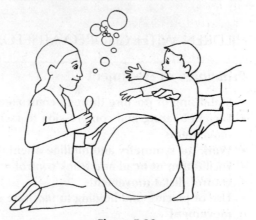

Figure 5.30
It should then be easier to bring him to standing. To reduce the flexor spasms, the therapist keeps pressure on the sacrum and gives some pressure down through the child's legs. He holds the child's arms forward to prevent any pull down

The following table gives more ideas about how to use key points of control.

Key point and tone-influencing pattern (TIP)	Likely effect
Child prone, head and neck extended, shoulder girdle retracted	Facilitates extension in rest of body
Child supine, head and neck flexed, shoulder girdle protracted	Reduces extensor spasticity
Inward rotation of shoulder with protraction of shoulder girdle	Reduces extensor spasticity and is useful in athetoids (used carefully) but in children with spasticity it increases flexor spasticity of neck, trunk and lower limbs
Outward rotation of shoulder with supination and elbow extension	Reduces flexion and increases extension in the rest of the body
Horizontal abduction of arms in outward rotation with supination and elbow extension	Reduces flexor spasticity. Facilitates opening of hand Facilitates abduction of the legs with outward rotation and extension if spine is also extended
Extension of arms backwards in prone, sitting or standing with spine extended	Reduces flexor spasticity. Has same effect as in horizontal abduction but easier to achieve when there is more spasticity
In sitting, prone or standing abduction of thumb with arm in outward rotation and supination	Facilitates opening of the fingers
Outward rotation of the legs in extension	Facilitates abduction of the hips and dorsiflexion of the ankles

CHILDREN WITH CHOREO-ATHETOSIS

Principles of treatment

- **Stabilising of posture through controlled stimulation and small ranges of movement**
- **Weight-bearing and compression to facilitate co-contraction and reduce involuntary movements**
- **Work for symmetry and midline orientation**
- **Facilitation of head and trunk control and proximal fixation to give child possibility to control distal movements**
- **Use of placing and holding to facilitate sustained tone and lead to better grading of movement**
- **Facilitation of reach and grasp**

The movements of children with choreo-athetosis are jerky and quick and in wide ranges. They lack stability, symmetry and grading of movement. In particular, they lack head and trunk control when they try to hold themselves up against gravity.

Without treatment, a child with athetosis is likely to be left in supine on the floor because there he is safe from falling. Propped in sitting, his extensor spasms are likely to put him in danger of falling backwards and hitting his head. It is very likely that he will hate being put in prone, because the poor stability in his trunk will make it difficult for him to lift his head, use his hands or move about. What usually happens is that he learns to push himself about in supine on the floor using his abnormal extension and good legs, while his arms push back uselessly in extension, outward rotation and retraction beside his head on the floor. This situation needs to be prevented if he is to develop any head and trunk control or any hand function. In fact, the first essential in treating children with athetosis is to get them up off the floor and put them in weight-bearing positions against gravity.

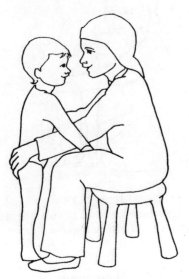

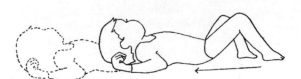

Figure 5.31
Pushing backwards along the floor is an easy way for an athetoid child to move about but it prevents him from using his hands or developing head control

Figure 5.32
Giving him opportunities to take weight on both arms and legs counteracts the child's pattern of moving in supine

Weight-bearing and compression through the child's limbs or trunk while in alignment, will steady the tone and facilitate the child to hold a posture. The more opportunities he gets to hold useful postures, the better able he will be to control the involuntary movements himself. While he is learning to do this, at first, however, he will not be able to tolerate much stimulation. The child with athetosis needs to build up tolerance to stimulation. During treatment, or while he is practising at home, he needs people to talk quietly to him so that he can begin to keep still in standing or sitting with weight-bearing and whatever support is necessary. His attention at this time should be focused on listening to a family member telling him a story or showing him pictures in a book. The book, or the person talking, must always be presented in the midline position so that the child does not turn his head and become ASYMMETRIC. As soon as he is steady enough, he can then start using one hand, with help, to manipulate a toy.

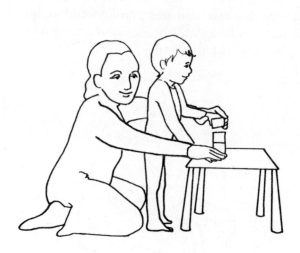

Figure 5.33
Therapist facilitates child to take weight on right arm while building tower with other hand

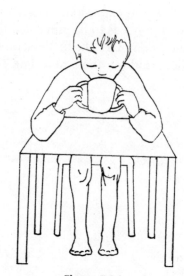

Figure 5.34
Once the child is able to take weight on his elbows, he may be able to drink with a two-handled cup by himself

As he learns to hold positions, the child must also learn to move, but without moving in wide ranges. If, for example, he becomes able to keep his head in midline and take weight through his arms in a supported sitting position, he could be facilitated to grasp a cup with both hands and bring it to his mouth. Or, perhaps he becomes able to be supported in standing so that he takes weight equally well on both feet. Most children with athetosis take weight well on one leg, while the other flexes and extends in a way that does not allow weight-bearing or even functional stepping. Once he can bear weight equally, he can be helped to take steps. This should be done in such a way that his body is in alignment and his head in midline. Many athetoid children learn to turn their heads to take steps. They turn their heads to the right to get extension and therefore weight-bearing on the right leg, and then they turn their heads to the left when they want to switch weight to the left.

It is very difficult for the child to take steps in a more normal way once he has learnt to do this. The constant head-turning also prevents him from being able to keep his head in midline and look where he is going.

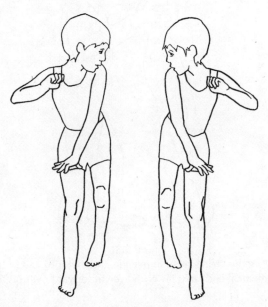

Figure 5.35
Child using head-turning to take steps. This reinforces his asymmetry

Children with athetosis, even more than other children, love to be on their feet and to be helped to take steps. This may be because their legs are often less affected than their arms and, as long as someone else holds and controls their trunk and arms, they know how to take steps. As treatment, helping a child with athetosis to walk is only useful if the child is kept in alignment and he is facilitated to take his full weight through his legs. Most families will help their child to walk by having him lean back against them while his legs take dancing steps way ahead of his body. This is not useful. The following pictures show some ways in which a good pattern of walking can be given. There are many other ways, depending on how the child's involuntary movements need to be controlled and how much support he needs in his trunk.

Enabling the child to *reach and grasp* is another essential part of the treatment of children with athetosis. For many children, just having both hands grasp a section of broom handle while keeping their heads in midline is a huge task. In order to learn to tolerate this, they must be placed in a position that is symmetrical and that does not allow them to throw themselves back into extension. Held in standing is probably the best position, but sitting in a chair with the hips kept firmly flexed is also good.

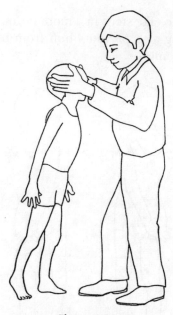

Figure 5.36
By holding the child's head in midline, the therapist can keep him
symmetrical and keep his body weight forward over his feet

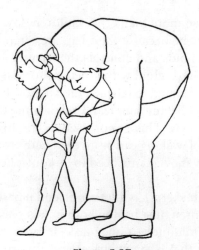

Figure 5.37
The therapist is preventing involuntary movements in the child's arms
at the same time as keeping her body weight forward and
giving pressure down through her legs

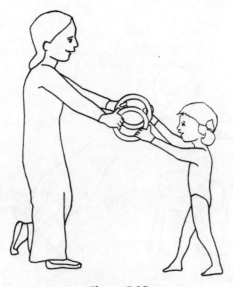

Figure 5.38
Holding onto the rings in this way keeps the child symmetrical and
allows the therapist to give more or less support as needed

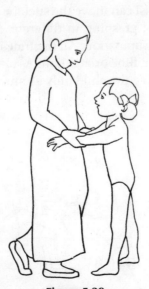

Figure 5.39
Holding the child's arms forward in extension gives symmetry
and therapist can keep the child's body weight forward

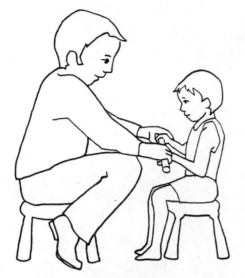

Figure 5.40
Having his head in midline and both hands
holding the stick can be difficult for an athetoid
child to tolerate

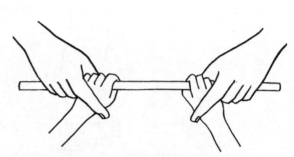

Figure 5.41
Detail showing how the therapist uses
his forefinger to hold the child's wrist in
extension while maintaining grasp

The broomstick is then placed in the child's hands, and the therapist facilitates bilateral
grasp with wrist extension and both of the child's arms in forward extension. Once he has
learnt to tolerate this, the therapist can move the stick in various directions to give the child
the sensori-motor experience of grasping in different directions. The grasp can also be
changed between PRONATION and supination. All the time the therapist must talk to the child
so that there is eye contact and midline orientation. As always with facilitation, the therapist
uses his hands sensitively, assisting the child only as much as necessary so that he learns to
control his own movements.

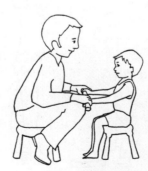

Figure 5.42
Once the child can tolerate having both hands grasping
with his elbows extended, he will be more ready to learn to reach and grasp

Although children with athetosis have strong extension in supine and in sitting, when they often throw themselves backwards uncontrollably, this extension is not useful for function. In order to acquire good trunk control, they need active extension against gravity. Prone would be the best position in which to acquire this, but most children with athetosis strongly object to being placed in prone. It may help such a child to be placed across his mother's knees; the mother should place one foot on a low stool so that the child is not horizontal. In this position, gravity will not have such a strong influence, and the child can be facilitated to raise his head and trunk and hold them in extension for a few seconds. As he becomes more able to hold the extension against gravity, the mother can, over some weeks, gradually lower her raised foot to make the child more horizontal. This is a good position in which to dress and undress the child.

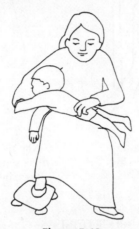

Figure 5.43
Using the prone position over the mother's knee for dressing and undressing helps the child to learn to tolerate being in prone and getting active extension of his head and trunk

In order to facilitate better *proximal fixation*, the therapist must use his hands on the child's pelvis, shoulder girdle or trunk to hold these proximal parts steady and in alignment and enable the child to have the experience of using his hands or legs in a useful way. Without this facilitation, the only way the child can fix himself proximally is to hold his trunk, shoulder girdle or pelvis in extreme positions, using his head to initiate the movement into the position. Since a child with athetosis almost always has his head turned to one side or the other and not in midline, the rest of his body is also asymmetrical. Treatment must therefore give him the experience of holding his shoulder girdle midway between protraction and retraction, of keeping his trunk midway between flexion and extension, and not side bending or rotating to either side. The pelvis also must be kept in alignment and not retracted or hitched up to either side. If all these parts are aligned, the child will be more likely to be able to maintain postures against gravity in preparation for learning fine motor skills.

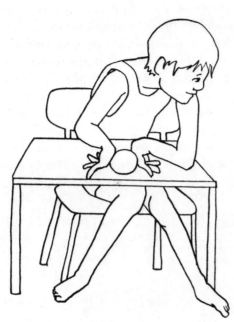

Figure 5.44
An athetoid child with poor trunk control
tries to fix himself using his arms and legs

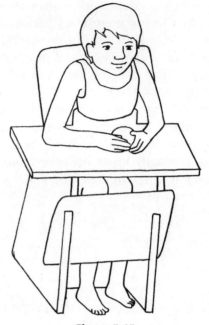

Figure 5.45
With his pelvis fixed by knee blocks, and his
trunk supported by a table, he can more easily
keep his head in midline and use his hands

CHILDREN WITH DYSTONIC ATHETOSIS

Principles of treatment

- **Analyse pattern of dystonic spasms and anticipate and prevent scoliosis**
- **Reduce frequency and duration of spasms**
- **Do not resist spasms**
- **Work for symmetry and midline orientation**
- **Facilitate head and trunk control, with particular attention to abdominal muscles, to counteract extensor spasms**
- **Keep stimulation low during treatment, and avoid frequent changes of position**
- **Use soft surfaces**

Children with dystonic athetosis can be the most difficult group of children with CP to treat. Their spasms are so strong and extreme that if they are resisted, either in handling or by fixing a child in positions, this can cause fractures or dislocations. We must therefore work to reduce them. Since the spasms mostly extend and rotate the upper trunk, treatment must aim to give the child the ability to come forward and take weight on his arms and hold his head in midline. This may be done in sitting on a stool with a table in front, or in prone over a soft roll, or—if both of these positions are too difficult—over two wedges to make an inverted V. But first it will probably be necessary to prepare the child, and to do this we must look at his trunk. Underlying the strong extensor spasms there may be a strong flexor pull in the opposite side of his trunk to which he turns his head, and until this is reduced it will be difficult to place the child in alignment. The pull down in the side of his trunk can be reduced by having him lie on the opposite side with his head on a small pillow and his knees a little bent up. Then, use your hands to elongate the uppermost side of his trunk, stretching out the muscles connecting his ribs and his pelvis. When you feel this loosen up, turn him slowly into prone over a small soft roll, and facilitate him to take weight on his forearms and lift his head. In this position he can gain better head control, and so can look at a toy or pictures in a book while you ensure he maintains alignment and weight-bearing on his forearms. Later, you can roll him carefully into supine with his knees bent up, then use his hands or wrists as key points of control to bring him up towards sitting, making sure that he uses his abdominals and not just his head and arms to pull. From this position, facilitate him to side sit to the side with the flexor pull, so that this is elongated. He may be able to take some weight on the hand on that side. After some time doing this, it may be easy to place him in sitting on the end of a bench, while you sit behind him keeping his shoulder girdle protracted and helping him to come forward and lean his arms on a padded table in front. Alternatively, it may be possible to get him up to standing, with support at his knees and hips and leaning forward onto a table to take weight on his forearms. Do this only as long as you can keep him in alignment and make sure there is no danger of him throwing himself and you off balance with a sudden spasm.

CHILDREN WITH ATAXIA

Principles of treatment

- Control postural tone by weight-bearing and joint compression
- Place and hold child in positions to facilitate co-contraction. Encourage child to take over so that you can release hold
- Use mobile weight-bearing and graded movements to change from one position to another
- Get selectivity of movement and independence of limbs from trunk
- Work for rotation around body axis
- Facilitate balance and protective reactions

A child with *ataxia* may fall over a lot, or he may have great difficulty in steadying himself and coordinating his movements in order to dress himself or hold a spoon to feed himself. Your assessment of the child with ataxia will show where he is failing in carrying out motor functions.

He falls over because the postural tone in his trunk and pelvis is inadequate, and also because he lacks grading of movement. He can't hold a spoon because his shoulder girdle does not hold his arm steady, and maybe also because he has intention tremor or overshoots.

To help him not to fall so much, he needs to be given the sensori-motor experience of recovering his balance when gravity threatens him. You will need to put him in positions where he is vulnerable but where he can be facilitated to accommodate to the threat of over-balancing. For example, hold one of his legs off the ground as he stands, and ask him to reach with each arm in turn in all directions. Don't let him fall, but don't support him so much that he is not stimulated enough to respond to prevent himself falling.

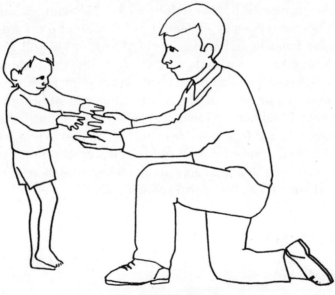

Figure 5.46
Facilitating balance reactions

Make him weight-bear on both arms while you lift his legs (*wheelbarrow walking*). If his tone is very low, you will need to support him above his knees. Get him to take steps so that he has to actively extend against gravity and rotate in his body axis (Figures 5.47 and 5.48).

Dressing and undressing should be a very important part of his treatment. Find the best positions for him so that he can use all the activities of dressing—sitting, standing, one leg raised, both arms raised overhead—to give him treatment at the same time as he is learning to be independent.

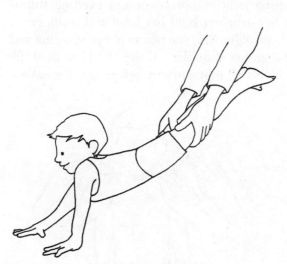

Figure 5.47
Wheelbarrow walking is a good way to
facilitate proximal (in this case trunk
and shoulder girdle) control

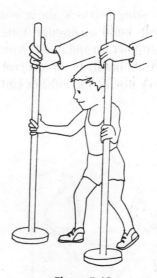

Figure 5.48
Learning to walk with long poles with broad
bases gives a child with ataxia confidence. The
therapist can give as much or as little support
as is necessary for the child not to fall

CHILDREN WITH HYPOTONIA

It is rare for a child to continue to have very low tone. Usually they change, sometimes quite quickly, to being athetoid, ataxic or spastic. If they do continue to have low tone, they are likely to also experience seizures and learning difficulties. In this case the main aim of treatment is to make them as active as possible and to find good positions in which they can be managed, that will not cause contractures and deformities.

You must be careful when stimulating young children with low tone, so that spasms don't suddenly take over. There is also the great danger that a child placed in positions that are appropriate for hypotonia may start to develop flexor contractures, and quite quickly might develop contractures, because those positions are not appropriate for flexor spasticity.

Principles of treatment

- **Work for sustained co-contraction**
- **Have the child work against gravity**
- **Use weight-bearing through all the limbs and in all positions**
- **Use sensory stimulation and joint compression**
- **Use vocalisation and laughter to build up tone**
- **Treat slowly—give child time to respond. Sustain positions to give child sensori-motor experience**
- **Be aware that low tone in young children can change to abnormally high tone or fluctuating tone**

The following pictures show a mother using joint compression and exciting stimulation to help build up enough tone to help her daughter hold her head and trunk erect. After jumping her up and down with her body in alignment, she places her in standing and uses her whole hands to tap downwards through her shoulders. If the child can hold the position very briefly, the mother can lift her hands off momentarily before tapping again.

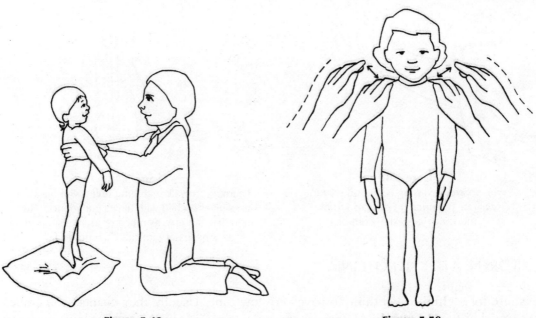

Figure 5.49
Bouncing on soft surface with child's head, trunk and legs in alignment facilitates co-contraction

Figure 5.50
Tapping through the child's shoulders with her body in alignment also facilitates co-contraction and helps her to hold herself upright for a short time

CHILDREN WITH MIXED CEREBRAL PALSY

The guiding principle in treating children with mixed CP is that you should treat what you find. In particular, look for how each child tries to compensate. For example, children with athetosis who continue to have poor postural control in their trunk, as time goes on very often develop flexor spasticity in their legs because they use their legs to give themselves fixation.

Children with ataxia sometimes show spasticity when they start to stand. They may stand with adduction and internal rotation of the hips to give themselves stability, but they will lack active hip extension.

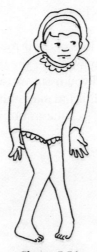

Figure 5.51
Ataxic child showing some spasticity
when she tries to balance in standing

If a child is hypotonic, stimulate him enough to give him some ability to hold himself up against gravity. If he shows signs of involuntary movements, make sure you work for head and trunk control and symmetry and midline orientation. If he shows signs of spasticity, use key points of control and TIPs to facilitate more normal patterns that will lead to independent functional activities.

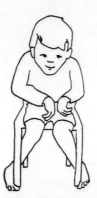

Figure 5.52
Athetoid boy trying to give himself fixation by hooking his feet around chair legs. This will increase the tone in his legs and may lead to flexor contractures. Treatment should aim to give him better trunk control

A FINAL WORD ON TREATMENT

This chapter has, I hope, given you an idea of the principles on which a treatment programme can be based. The examples given may work for the child you are treating, or they may not. They are only examples. In each child you treat, you will have to work out what is the most important thing to achieve for that child, and make sure your treatment is aimed at achieving that. If it does not, then change your treatment, but stick to the principles.

Chapter 6

Child, family and therapist
working as a team

THIS chapter will look at ways in which therapists and families can best relate to each other and work together. I have chosen to talk about families rather than parents because, very often, the whole extended family can work in partnership with the therapist to help the child function better at home. Although in most cases mothers are the main carers, sometimes a brother or sister has more time than a mother to use play to help the child to function better. Sometimes an aunt or uncle can persuade a child to do more difficult activities. This is not a criticism of the mother; rather, it is a realisation that a mother's relationship with her child may not al-ways be compatible with her working with him as a therapist does. A child looks to his mother for protection and comfort. Exercises may challenge him and make him feel insecure, and he may feel confused if it is his mother who instigates such a feeling.

Another reason for choosing to work with the wider family is that the attitude of the family as a whole can have a huge impact on how the mother feels about her child, and even how she handles him in his daily care. This makes it important for therapists to seek opportunities to work with other members of the family as well as the mother.

This chapter is divided into two parts. Part 1 deals with the issue of partnership between therapist and family. Part 2 deals with how therapy can be carried out as part of daily care.

PART 1: HOW THERAPISTS CAN BE GOOD PARTNERS

Research has shown that, no matter how expert the treatment, physiotherapy or occupational therapy alone cannot make significant improvement in the child's condition. There has to be carry-over from the treatment into the child's everyday life. As therapists, it is our responsibility not only to help families understand this, but also to enable them to put it into practice.

This poses a problem for many therapists. Instead of treating children ourselves and using our skills to enable them to do things they could not do before, we are being asked to pass on our hard-earned knowledge and skills to every family, no matter what its circumstances or level of education may be. Many therapists feel that by doing this they are undermining their own professional status.

I think we should look at it like this: as therapists we have the knowledge and skills that enable us to assess, and then design a programme for, children of all ages with all types of CP. We are passing on to each family the understanding and skill that they need to enable them to work with their own unique child. By doing this we are planting the seeds from which an effective partnership will grow and bear fruit. And there is the even more compelling reason that if we don't teach the families what we know about their children, we cannot bring about any lasting improvement in their condition.

So, as well as being therapists, we must also be teachers and trainers. To some extent we have to be social workers too, because before we can work with a family we have to understand a good deal about them. We need to know

- what their attitude to the child and his disability is,
- what their home situation is like,
- what coping mechanisms they have,
- what capacity for learning they have, and
- what relevant knowledge, skills and insight they have.

We have to learn the skills that enable us to gather this information from the family, without seeming to be inquisitive. This requires us to develop a friendly way of behaving and interacting with them. At the same time, they have to feel able to trust us to keep the information they give us totally confidential. They have to feel safe, that the secrets they share with us will not be used for anything except the benefit of their child. I think there are very few therapists who have been trained to do these things as part of their basic education. They are expected to learn 'on the job', often without any role models. This is a very difficult thing to do. It means making a fundamental change in how you see yourself as a therapist. In order to do this it might help to look at some recent material that has been written on the roles of professional people (such as doctors, lawyers, therapists, accountants).

Reading the research, as a professional, can be depressing. Professional people, it seems, are not very popular! This attitude to professionals is reflected in the findings of a number of research projects that have shown that patients and clients feel oppressed by the power they feel professionals exert over them. In his book, *Challenging the Professions: Frontiers for Rural Development* (London, 1993), Robert Chambers describes how rural communities in developing countries were the very last people to be consulted when the economists and engineers were planning a project. After the project had been completed it was discovered that it was quite inappropriate for local needs. If only the professionals had consulted the local people in time, a lot of money and effort would have been saved. Situations like this have encouraged people planning services to feel they can manage without professionals. In some countries, community-based rehabilitation programmes are being run without therapists, because the planners say that therapists bias the programme towards the *medical model* when what local communities need is the *social model*.

The *medical model* tends to focus on the individual as a patient, attempting to make him or her as 'normal' as possible. Control of rehabilitation is solely in the hands of medical experts. Success or failure is seen only in terms of how the medical programme enables the disabled person to conform to what society regards as normal. Those who cannot achieve this 'normality' are considered failures by society, and of course the therapists will also feel they have failed.

The *social model* tends to imagine that impairment is not the real obstacle. Efforts are focused on encouraging the community to accept the person just as he or she is, and on adapting structures within the community to accommodate to disabled people's needs. Control of these efforts is much more in the hands of the community and of disabled people (or their families) themselves.

The *balanced model* is the model accepted by the World Health Organisation. It combines and integrates good quality individual rehabilitation with efforts to bring about social inclusion for the child and his or her family. In this model the evaluation of needs and the search for solutions are shared between all concerned in a cooperative way.

I have seen the failure of the medical model in many of the different countries where I have taught. In these countries I often hear therapists complain about parents: 'They don't care enough about their children to work with them,' 'They are not educated enough to understand the importance of treatment,' or 'Parents are lazy, they just want us to do all the work.' I believe what happens is this: parents come to therapists in the hope and expectation of a medical cure for their child's condition. They are likely to be very worried and depressed about their child and they are not likely to be impressed by a cure that comes in the form of exercises that may seem just like playing. And so either they do not comply, or they carry out the exercises but without any faith in their value. After some time they lose hope that even these efforts can make any difference.

The therapist, on the other hand, has a huge number of children to treat. It is tempting to concentrate time and effort on those families who listen easily to advice, who understand that the exercise programme will help and who have enough time and energy to give to their children. The therapist thinks, 'It's not my fault if people don't listen to my advice,' and he or she takes less and less time and trouble over those families who seem not to care. In the end they stop coming, and the child is left untreated at home. In places where there are few therapists and a large number of children to treat, this happens to the majority of children. Only a few parents are able to act on the therapists' advice.

The social model may be successful in giving the family and the child a much better environment in which to function. Families, however will very often worry that their child is not having opportunities, to learn to walk, for instance. This is because no one involved with the programme has the necessary expertise to advise them as to how they can best help with this. Without good therapy, it is certain that the dangers of contractures and deformities will be much greater.

Padmani Mendis in her paper on community-based rehabilitation (CBR) wrote that when physiotherapists (or well-trained rehabilitation workers) were involved in a programme the output, in terms of both quality and coverage, was greater. So there is recognition that expertise is necessary. It is not, however, the existence of the expertise that is in question, it is the way in which this expertise is delivered to people with disabilities, or to their families, that can be a problem. In his book *Disability, Liberation and Development*, Peter Coleridge has written in a very sensitive and telling way about the relationship between therapists and people with disabilities. He says, 'nobody is arguing for fewer professionals: let us be very clear about that. They are vital. What is at issue is the underlying attitude they bring to the job. What disabled people want is to join with professionals in formulating policy on rehabilitation and then to work with them to implement it. This is an exciting positive process which in no way detracts from or undermines the importance of the professional task; on the contrary, it enhances it.' The 'underlying attitude' he is talking about is the way in which therapists tend to think of the people they work with as 'cases' or 'patients' rather than people. A 'case' is something to be cured and made 'normal'. What a disabled person wants is to be seen as a whole person. This includes these children and their families. To be able to work with a family successfully, the therapist needs to

- include the family and the child in the planning of the child's programme,
- help the family and child to accept what cannot be cured, and
- always work towards functional goals that the child or family have chosen and that help towards social integration.

We must give up the idea that in some way we are in control of the children and their families. We are there to serve their needs, and we can only do this by understanding those needs and by using our knowledge and expertise to help the family to meet them in their own way.

One of the most important tasks we have is helping the family to come to terms with their child's condition. Both therapists and parents have the difficult task of realising that therapy can give good but limited results. Through therapy some children will become independent, and perhaps able to earn a living, others will become partially independent, and still others can only be helped by making them easier to look after. This can be a painful and difficult truth to accept. The process of acceptance will be slow and costly, but without it there will be only disappointment and despair.

There are personal qualities that we can develop, in the same way that we develop handling skills, to help us in this difficult task. These qualities are: being able to

- listen and show you understand,
- allow family to participate as equal partners,
- give information clearly, and
- teach handling skills.

Listening and understanding

These skills need to be thought about and practised. Not being ready to listen is one of the most frequent criticisms families make about some professionals.

We need first to think about what makes for good listening. Think about the following list of elements of good listening and ask yourself how many of them you employ in your listening to families.

- *Putting aside your own opinions.* Don't judge parents and don't allow your own assumptions to interfere with your ability to pay attention and absorb information from them.

- *An open posture.* Does the way you are sitting show that you are interested? Sitting with crossed legs and folded arms, for example, can make you look tense and impatient. Your posture should show that you are relaxed but attentive.

- *Eye contact.* The amount of eye contact you make will vary from one culture to another. The important thing is to make sure that you make eye contact in the right way to give the parent the feeling that you are taking in what they are saying.

- *Facial expression.* Again, this will vary from one culture to another, but the way you change your facial expression as you listen should reflect your interest and sympathy. It should never reflect disapproval or criticism. Even if a mother tells you that sometimes she feels total rejection for her child, it is not appropriate for you to be critical of this feeling. Rather, it is necessary for you to show that you accept and are trying to understand her feelings and you are glad she is able to tell you about them.

- *Attentive silence.* It is important to leave enough silence for the parent to be encouraged to go on talking.

- *Giving the right encouragement.* Small acknowledgements from time to time that you have heard and understood what the parent has said—but don't interrupt the flow of speech—are good encouragement. For example, you could say things like, 'I see,' or 'Really,' or even just 'Mm-hm.'

- *Asking open questions.* These are questions that have to be answered at length. They cannot be answered with 'Yes' or 'No.' For example, you could ask a parent, 'How does your child spend her day at home?' or 'How did you feel when you first learnt that your little boy had cerebral palsy?'

- *Giving feedback.* Letting the parent know that you have understood by summarising the answers. For example, 'I see, so your little boy spends most of his day lying on the floor but you sometimes prop him up on a chair.' Sometimes it is difficult for a parent to describe a situation, and then you could ask further questions to help them give you a clearer picture. For example, 'I'm sorry I don't quite understand, do you mean…?'

It is important to be aware, though, that getting a parent to talk, and listening in an open, accepting way can cause uncomfortable feelings. The parent may feel he or she is taking up too much of the therapist's time, or feel frustrated because the therapist is not coming up with an instant solution to their problem. The therapist, on the other hand, may be very tempted to abandon the quiet listening approach and to come in too quickly with solutions and advice. The opportunity may then be missed to hear everything the parents want to say, and the therapist will not have the full picture of how they manage as a family.

Coming to an agreement for action

According to the medical model, the therapist decides on a programme for the child and gives the family a list of exercises they must do with the child at home. This seldom works. A better approach is one of equal participation of the therapist and the family in the problem-solving process.

The therapist and the family each come to the situation with a very different point of view. The therapist comes with the responsibility for achieving the best rehabilitation for the child; he will be thinking about how to prevent contractures and deformities and how to enable the child to be as independent as possible and to achieve the best quality of life. The family, on the other hand, have the responsibility for the child as a whole and for the family as a whole. A deal has to be struck that accommodates both these perspectives.

Forming a partnership is a process which must start with open and honest sharing of information between parent and therapist. As can be seen from the diagram on the facing page, this leads to a shared definition of the problem. From the parent's point of view, the problem may be the other demands on their time and effort besides what they have to give to their child. From the therapist's point of view, the problem may be what will happen if the child is not given at least a minimum amount of the parent's time. What is important, if the partnership is to be successful, is that each one understands the other's point of view.

What family and therapist each has to bring to the partnership

What the family has to bring	What the therapist has to bring
• Knowledge of the child as a person learnt from the day-to-day experience of giving care	Knowledge of how CP interferes with a child's ability to hold postures and to move normally. Ability to assess what is interfering with the child's ability to function
• Awareness of how the child is perceived in the family	• Experience of how other families have learnt to perceive children in a more positive light
• Knowledge of the support that is available and can be called upon, from family members and the local community	• Knowledge of what can be done to improve the child's functional ability, and also what dangers of contractures and deformities are present if the child does not receive good treatment and handling
• Lifelong commitment to the child	• Commitment to offering professional service to child and family
• Time given to caring for the child—dressing, toilet care, feeding	• Ability to make the kind of relationship with the family that will enable them to work effectively with the child
• Own coping strategies for dealing with hardship and stress	• Ability to adapt the treatment programme to fit the family circumstances
• Knowledge of local environment within which the child can find opportunities to play and interact socially with other children	• Ability to keep good records and to be able to demonstrate to the family how goals have been reached and improvement achieved

Once both partners have accepted each other's definition of the problem, both of them can suggest solutions. The parents' solutions are given equal weight to the therapist's solutions as long as the therapist's reasons for doing things in a certain way are understood and accepted, and as long as the parents' reasons for perhaps *not* being able to carry out certain activities at home are also understood and accepted. Then the decision to carry out the programme can be made and implemented in true partnership.

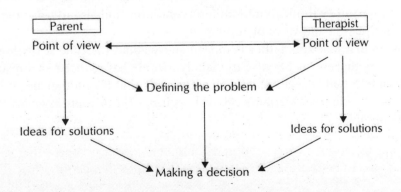

Case study

Mariam is 2 years old and has cerebral palsy. She is mainly floppy but she is beginning to show some involuntary movements. She needs to be placed in good sitting and standing positions so that she can develop some postural control in an upright position. If she does not get this experience she will start pushing herself around the floor on her back and this will reduce her chances of developing any hand function and of, later, learning to walk.

Mariam's family are extremely poor. She lives with her three brothers and two sisters in very cramped conditions. Her father is a small farmer. Her mother has been bringing Mariam to see the physiotherapist for several weeks, but it is clear that she has not been carrying out the home programme.

The physiotherapist decides to take a whole session just talking with Mariam's mother to try to negotiate a decision on how to solve the problem. At first, Mariam's mother is very defensive, and tries to insist that she does work hard with her daughter at home. The physiotherapist does not challenge this but instead points out that it must be very hard for her to find time and energy to do any extra work at home. She sympathises wholeheartedly with her and shows that she understands what life must be like for her. Mariam's mother starts to cry and then she pours out all her concerns. Her husband gets angry because he feels she shouldn't take time to work with Mariam. He thinks Mariam will never be of any use and she should just leave her without much attention. Also, before Mariam was born, her mother used to sell some vegetables to supplement the family income. Now she can't do this any more because she doesn't have time. She is also too tired and depressed.

The physiotherapist realises that the mother alone cannot deal with these problems. She tells her this and then suggests that, if possible, on her next visit, she bring along her husband and any other member of the family who might be willing and able to help, Mariam's mother is greatly relieved to be told that the responsibility for her daughter is not hers alone.

The following week, Mariam's mother manages to bring her husband with her, and also her husband's mother. The physiotherapist finds a quiet place where they can all discuss the problem together. She then asks some open questions to the husband and mother-in-law to find out what they think about Mariam's condition, and also to learn more about the whole family's situation and ways of coping.

She discovers that Mariam's father is indeed angry about the time his wife spends with Mariam. He hints that this is because the family income has reduced as a result of her no longer being able to sell vegetables. She also discovers that his mother has time to spend, but that she has the idea that Mariam's case is hopeless. (*The therapist is giving the family the chance to talk openly.*)

Problem defined

- **Family's point of view: No use working on a hopeless case**
- **Therapist's point of view: Without work at home, the child's case will be less hopeful**

The therapist lets the family know that she understands completely what they have told her, and that she does not in any way judge or condemn their feelings and attitudes. She then tells them that she needs them to understand her point of view about Mariam. She needs them, first, to know that many children who are floppy like Mariam can learn to walk in time if they are given some good handling early in their lives. Second, she tells them that they need to understand that if Mariam is not given opportunities to be in standing and sitting, she will be much more difficult to handle and look after as she grows bigger. (*The therapist expresses her opinions clearly.*)

She tells them that she will help them to find ways to put Mariam in standing and sitting that will not make extra work for them. She asks them if they have any ideas about how to solve the problem of who will help Mariam's mother in carrying out Mariam's care. She explains that if Mariam is dressed in the right position, carried about in the right position and encouraged to use her hands when playing, this will be her treatment. If everybody who handles her does these things in the right way, then in three months' time Mariam will, very likely, be sitting alone at least for a minute or two. (*The therapist puts forward some helpful suggestions.*)

The idea that there is hope for Mariam to improve and that a definite goal can be achieved is very encouraging for the family. The grandmother immediately says she will help for an hour or two every day so that Mariam's mother can start growing vegetables for the market again. Her father says that he is willing to help her play whenever he is home, and that he will encourage the other children in the family to do the same.

Decision reached by both therapist and family

- **Each one is happy that what has been decided is possible and likely to be effective**
- **Participation increases responsibility**

These suggestions are, largely, the family's own ideas. They are not imposed on them by the physiotherapist. Therefore, the family will be more likely to carry them out.

Before they leave, the physiotherapist shows all of them how best to lift and carry Mariam, and also shows them some satisfying games to play with her in a good position. She tells them that next time they come, they will discuss together what kind of chair and standing frame they will find most useful so that Mariam could be placed in sitting and standing.

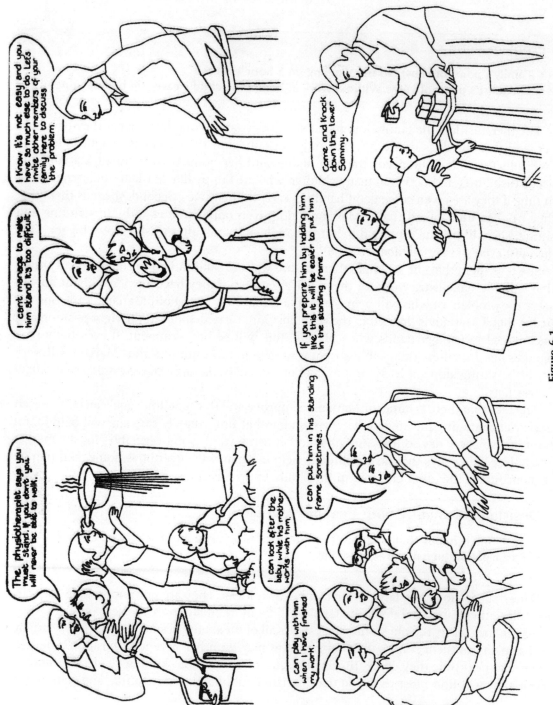

Figure 6.1

Being able to give information

Different people grasp the information they are given in different ways. Some people need to have the information written down, others understand better if the information is explained verbally and demonstrated. As therapists, we need to find out how each family member we are working with can best understand the information we are giving.

We have to also remember that often parents are feeling too upset to take in any information. When a mother is in a state of shock and disbelief that her child is disabled, the only information she can take in is something that gives her hope and comfort. A way of carrying her child or positioning her that is clearly making the child less stiff or less floppy will be the kind of information that she might be able to understand and remember. She will also be more able to accept information given to her by someone she trusts, someone whom she knows understands her feelings and respects her as a person. In her vulnerable state she may think that the world has a right to reject her. As therapists, we are responsible for building up her confidence in herself as a person and as a mother. We can do this by giving her only as much information as she can take in and by helping her to act on that information.

Families are not in a state of shock all the time, however. They manage in many ways to come to terms with their situation, and we must support them as they learn to cope. As Mariam's case study demonstrated, giving information to the family as a whole, rather than just one member, is a good way of doing this. If the mother is the only person being given the information, she has the extra burden of acting on that information alone and of trying to convince other family members that this is the right thing to do. They may not be convinced, and then the therapist will have caused divisions in the family.

It is strange how we human beings decide which information to act upon and which not! For example, we know it is bad for us to be overweight, to smoke, not to exercise or to lift things in the wrong way. But do we, truthfully, always act upon this knowledge? It is interesting to reflect upon why we don't. We are more often tempted to do the things that are bad for us when we are depressed and our self-esteem is low. The same is true for families with children who have CP. They know they should do 'exercises' with their children, but they are tempted to neglect this difficult duty because they don't believe they can make a good job of it. Our first duty, then, is to convince them that they can, and that it will make a difference. The information we give to the family must be just enough for them to understand exactly what we are asking them to do and why we are asking them to do it. For example, 'If you place your child in a standing frame for 10 minutes every day, he will start to be able to balance better in sitting.' The information should also be linked to some aspect of the child's lack of ability that the family have expressed worries about. If the activity we are asking them to do is directly linked to overcoming a problem they are concerned about, they will be more likely to be motivated to carry out that activity.

Choosing short-term goals

A key to giving families hope is being able to choose short-term goals and inform the family about them. This means being able to say that some measurable improvement will happen if the programme agreed between the family and the therapist is carried out.

An example might be of a child who pushes back into extension with any stimulation, and whose mother is having problems carrying him or leaving him in any position except supine on the floor. The programme negotiated with the family is that the child will be carried in a sitting position with no pressure against his head, and that he will be placed in a prone standing frame for 15 minutes twice a day. He will have one meal while standing in the standing frame. He will spend as much of the rest of the day as possible in a side lying position with toys suspended so that he can touch them with his hands. The measurable improvement at the end of six weeks of this programme might be that the child can hold his head erect for one minute while he is held in a sitting position. This small piece of improvement may not seem very impressive. However, if it has been predicted by the therapist and the programme has been faithfully carried out by the family, all concerned may be justified in feeling a sense of real achievement and be encouraged to move on to the next step.

Some families find it helpful to have a notebook in which the programme is written down and the goal they are working towards described. They might like to place a tick on a chart for every part of the programme they carry out. Over a period of a year or more, they will be pleased to look back at the number of goals they have achieved. They will also have built up a high level of confidence in their own ability to bring about improvement in the child's condition.

Example of page in home programme notebook

Date	Placed in standing	Placed side lying	Ate whole meal in standing
1/6	✓	✓	✗
2/6	✓	✓✓	✗
3/6	✓✓	✓✓	✗
4/6	✓	✓✓✓	✗
5/6	✓✓	✓✓	✓
6/6	✓✓	✓✓✓	✗
7/6	✓✓	✓✓	✓

The following table could be written at the back of the same notebook so that the family can see the slow but steady progress their child is making.

Of course, it is not easy to accurately predict the child's improvement. It takes experience to know what is possible and what might be too ambitious. If you find you are being overoptimistic in your predictions, try to choose a slightly longer timeframe or a less difficult task. The important thing is to offer realistic hope without giving too definite promises.

Example of page in home programme notebook

Short-term goal	When set	When achieved
Sammy will be able to hold his head erect for one minute while he is held in sitting	3/6/99	18/7/99
Sammy will be able to lift his head and hold it up for one minute while lying face down over a roll	18/7/99	2/9/99
Sammy will be able to balance alone in sitting on the floor for one minute	2/9/99	20/10/99

Exceptionally difficult relationships

With most families, it is possible to form a working relationship that benefits the child. Sometimes the therapist has to accept that a family cannot do as much with the child as she would like, and she has to adapt her programme to suit the family's needs and abilities. At other times the family has to listen to the advice of the therapist so that they can make an informed choice about how to manage their child. As long as there is a close relationship between therapist and family, these issues can usually be resolved.

In some instances, however, it becomes difficult to the point of being impossible to work with a family. This usually comes about because the family is under some severe strain other than that of having a disabled child. The family may be living in dire poverty, or one of the parents may be suffering from mental illness. Perhaps the family have lived through terrible experiences that have left them traumatised.

On the other hand it must be recognised that, sometimes, therapists themselves become stressed and overburdened. Many hard-working, conscientious therapists burn out because they are overwhelmed by the emotional and physical stress of the job they do. In such cases it may help all concerned if the therapist takes a few weeks' break from therapy. During this time off, the therapist should have the opportunity to discuss her problems with a colleague or with a programme manager. Perhaps the family would do better with a new therapist for a while, or perhaps the colleague or programme manager could negotiate with the family so that a different member of the family works with the therapist and child for a while.

While everything possible must be tried for the sake of the child, sometimes cooperation fails and the relationship between the family and the therapist is one of disagreement and even hostility. Even so, it may not be necessary to give up on a family completely. It maybe possible to get back into a relationship with them when their circumstances or access to resources changes, or when they recognise their child's need for therapy. That is why it is important, even with the unfriendliest family, to try to part without harsh words so that the door is left open for a return to cooperation.

Partnership with children

So far, this chapter has concentrated on working in partnership with the adults in a child's family. It should, however, be every therapist's ambition to draw children themselves into the process of working in partnership. It is easy to underestimate how much even very young children understand. It can cause serious distress to a child and his family if a therapist talks about the child as if he is not there or as if he can't understand, when in fact he understands well. This is particularly true of children who have difficulty speaking. It is a wise therapist who, from the first contact with a child, talks to that child in a manner that conveys a readiness to be close and to understand what the child might want to communicate.

Above all, the therapist should understand every child's fundamental need to be able to play. Their cerebral palsy, and perhaps also their learning difficulty, may be preventing them from using play in the way that normal children do, to explore the world around them and to make some sense of it. The programme the therapist decides on for each child must take this into account, and the child must be helped to play in a way that is satisfying. In order to engage children in active participation in their treatment, it is essential to choose play activities at the right level and within the intellectual capability of the child. Once the child realises that his therapist can help him to play in the way that he so longs for, he will be more ready to cooperate and work with the therapist to also achieve some of the therapist's objectives. The therapist may want the child to be placed in standing, perhaps, or balance in sitting, but the child just wants to play. Both can achieve their objectives if the therapist sets the scene in just the right way.

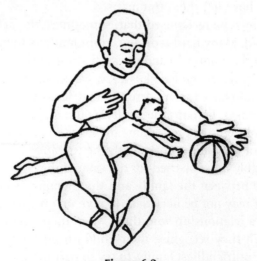

Figure 6.2
The child is playing, while the therapist is looking for good active extension

From a very early stage the therapist can communicate to the child, for example, how it is good to be in standing: how he can see more, how tall it makes him and how strong it makes his legs. Later, when the child can understand a lot, it is very important to explain clearly why exercises are important.

Many children are capable of taking responsibility for some of their own treatment from an early age. But this can only happen under certain conditions. The first of these conditions is that the therapist and the child's family believe the child is capable of taking responsibility, and they communicate this to him. The second is that the child feels capable and is proud of this. Choosing the right task to start the child working in this way is obviously crucial. It must be a task that the child understands to be useful. An example might be a child who spends some hours sitting at a school desk every day. To counteract this, when he comes home he does some active hip and knee extension in standing. This is a self-disciplined way of working. The child knows it helps him and he trains himself to do it. It would help if he knows of other children who work in the same way. Children who have learnt to be self-disciplined will take a great load off their parents' shoulders. They will avoid the usual ineffectual nagging that parents fall back on when things are difficult, and they will be prepared for a lifetime of understanding their condition and taking responsibility for making the best of their lives.

All this achievement, however, depends on the therapist communicating in a good way with the family and the child. It depends on him choosing the right tasks for the child to take responsibility for, and finally it depends on him being able to teach the child to carry out the exercises in the right way so that the child feels good about his achievements and motivated to continue.

PART 2: THERAPY AS PART OF DAILY CARE

In the chapter on treatment I touched on a few ways of carrying and positioning children. This chapter will cover more fully the different ways in which the handling and placing of children can be made easier for families. It will also show how everyday activities can be actual treatment for a child.

It is likely that a child will have to be lifted and carried around at some point in the day. He or she may also have to be dressed and undressed, bathed and taken to the toilet, and in between left in one position or another that is safe. Some families are so stressed and busy that they may not be able to do anything more with their child than take care of these basic needs. If we can at least help them to carry out these activities in a way that is easier for them and of benefit to the child, we won't have to feel the child is getting no treatment.

The most important thing of all to teach the whole family is how to lift the child. Many people lift a child up from the floor as in the following illustration.

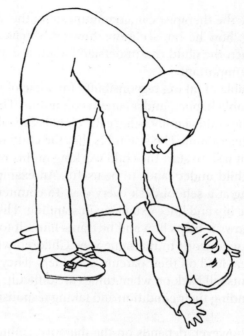

Figure 6.3
Lifting like this puts a strain on the lifter's back

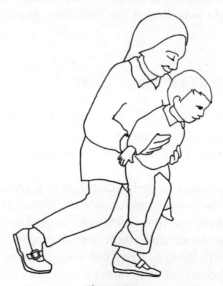

Figure 6.4
Holding the child close to the lifter's body and
using her leg muscles to lift protects her back from strain

Lifting with straight legs and a bent back puts all the strain on the small muscles of the lifter's spine. In time, these muscles are damaged and back pain can become chronic. The secret to protecting the lifter's back is to lift in such a way that the legs, rather than the back, take the strain. The child must be held close to the lifter's body, not at arm's length, and the back should be kept straight while the hips and knees bend.

Most parents tend to handle children too quickly. It may be necessary to take a good deal of time to explain to them that if they handle their children more slowly and give them time to respond, they will be helping them to develop. As a child is lifted up in stages from the floor, for instance, she will try to hold her head steady in each stage. If she is just scooped up, there is no time for her to begin to take control. Another example is when a child is dressed quickly and given no time to try to push his arm into a sleeve or lift one foot to place in his trousers.

Teaching handling skills is an art. Often therapists try to teach families how to handle their children just by demonstrating, and parents may be embarrassed about trying out the skill in front of the therapist. Without specific training, however, it is not possible to expect a parent to change from the way they have always handled their child to a wholly new way. Success will come only through step-by-step teaching of parents and family while giving them constant reassurance that they are doing a good job. But they will only be doing a good job if the therapist has chosen the right task for them to do and has been a patient and skilful teacher.

As you teach people these handling skills, try to remember how you felt the last time you had to learn to do something difficult. When you were a student, learning to carry out passive movements or set up electrotherapy treatment, how easy was it to learn when your teacher was watching every move? When he was patient and encouraging, was it easier to learn than when he was critical or when his body language made him seem so?

Possible ways of carrying a child*

Type of CP	One way of carrying small child	Alternate way for small child	Large child
Severe spastic extended child	Push back is prevented by holding hips in flexion and not supporting head	Prevents abnormal push back and facilitates postural control of head	Flexion and abduction of hips prevents abnormal push back
Severe spastic flexed child	Child is held in good extension and encouraged to actively lift head	Child is held in good extension and encouraged to actively lift head	Arms are prevented from pulling down into flexion. Head and trunk encouraged to actively extend
Moderate spastic quadriplegia	To prevent flexor spasticity and facilitate active extension	To prevent adduction and internal rotation of hips and facilitate postural control of head and trunk	To inhibit pull down in arms
Spastic diplegia	To prevent adduction and internal rotation of hips and facilitate postural control of head and trunk	To prevent adduction and internal rotation of hips and facilitate postural control of head and trunk	To prevent adduction and internal rotation of hips and facilitate postural control of head and trunk

*These are only suggested ways for carrying children. If they work to help the mother carry her child more easily or to help the child to have better postural control, use them. If not, try some other way.

(continued)

Possible ways of carrying a child (*continued*)

Type of CP	One way of carrying small child	Alternate way for small child	Large child
Hemiplegia	Hemi side facing forward helps head turning to affected side	To inhibit retraction of hemi side	Child walks alone but, if insecure, hold hemi hand
Athetoid	To facilitate symmetry and postural control of head	To facilitate symmetry and postural control of head	Held in alignment for symmetry and postural control of head
Athetoid with dystonic spasm	To prevent extensor spasm and encourage active extension	Hips held flexed to prevent push back	To prevent extensor spasm and encourage active extension
Floppy child	To give sensori-motor experience of upright position and facilitate postural control of head	To give sensori-motor experience of upright position	To facilitate holding head erect

Suggested positions in which to dress children

Type of CP	Baby	Older child	More able child
Severe spastic extended child	Prevents extensor spasticity facilitates active extension	Mother's legs (one behind pelvis, one over child's legs) gives stability and leaves hands free	Child helps in dressing. Own active flexion prevents push back into extension
Severe spastic flexed child	Movement of mother's legs helps prevent flexor spasticity	Encourages active extension of head and trunk from stable base	Child helps in dressing. Own active extension prevents flexor spasticity
Moderate spastic quadriplegia	Encourages active extension in trunk and movement of arms away from trunk	Mother's legs (one behind pelvis, other over child's legs) keep child's hips flexed and her hands free to help child dress	Mother's legs (one behind pelvis, other over child's legs) keep child's hips flexed and her hands free to help child dress
Athetoid	Flexed hips prevent push back. Neck cushion gives possibility of head in midline	Encourages active head raising and symmetry	Gives proximal fixation and possibility of dressing self

(continued)

Suggested positions in which to dress children (*continued*)

Type of CP	Baby	Older child	More able child
Athetoid with dystonic spasm	Hip flexion prevents push back. Neck cushion gives symmetry	Prevents extensor spasms. Facilitates holding head and trunk in mid-position	Mother's legs (one behind pelvis, the other over child's legs) give proximal fixation so child can actively help
Hemiplegia	Use opportunity to get head turning to hemi side. Put hemi limbs in first	Mother sits at hemi side. Prevents neglect of hemi side and unequal weight-bearing	Using hemi hand with help while holding on with unaffected hand
Floppy child	Possibility of seeing own limbs and helping in dressing	Good position to facilitate head raising	Mother's legs (one behind pelvis, the other over child's legs) give support so child can be active in trunk and arms

It is not possible to describe the exact dressing position that is best for every kind of child. These tables are meant only to give guidelines. Try to remember that weight-bearing on arms is very important and functionally useful for all children. If you can use dressing to facilitate this then try to include it in your instructions to the family. Rotation in the body axis is also very useful and helps to reduce spasticity. It is often easy to facilitate rotation while the child is prone over the mother's knees. In a more able child, shifting weight from one side to the other, to lift one leg and put on a sock for instance, is another way to facilitate rotation.

Before teaching family members about dressing the child, however, do ask them to show you how they do it themselves and ask what difficulties they have with it. If you see something going very wrong (for example, the child becoming very asymmetric) then gently suggest, show them and let them try a different way and explain why you think it might help the child. As a general rule, choose only one thing at a time to change so that the family is not overwhelmed with new instructions.

Chapter 7

Useful equipment at a treatment centre and at home

WE use equipment for children with CP to give them opportunities to be in positions that will help them to develop better postural control, better hand function and better communication and interaction with people around them. The equipment supports the child in positions that he cannot assume and maintain himself, and frees the therapist's hands to work with different parts of his body. At home, the equipment is used for the child to gain the experience of new positions on a daily basis, for half an hour or so at a time. It should be able to support the child almost as well as we could with our hands. Support from equipment can never be dynamic, as our hand support is, but it allows the child to hold a position longer than we or the family have time for and allows him more freedom, independence and control.

EQUIPMENT TO BE USED AT A THERAPY CENTRE

Floor mats
Firm, padded, washable floor mats should be used when treating all young children. They will feel safe on these and also be free to move.

Medical plinths (padded tables)
Low plinths (not more than 45 cm in height) are useful for older children, and also for working with children in standing and some sequences of movement. The medical plinths that are normally used in physiotherapy departments are too high and too narrow for young children. They serve to reinforce the perception that therapy is a medical cure: that the therapist is going to 'do something' to the child while the mother sits apart, detached from the procedure. Most children, when they are put in lying on a high medical plinth, are aware of this and become fearful. These plinths should therefore not be used for children.

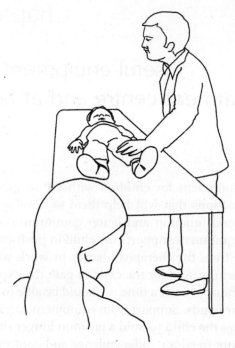

Figure 7.1
A high plinth is unfriendly to mother and child

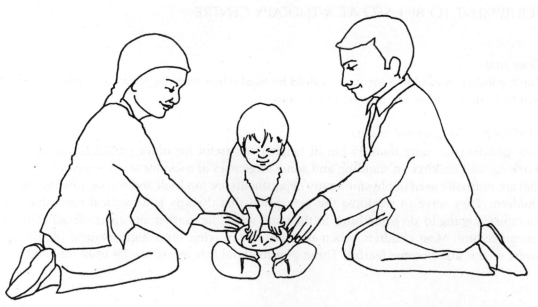

Figure 7.2
Floor mats are more natural

Rolls (firm foam rubber cylinders covered in plastic)
Rolls are useful during treatment because they lift one part of the child's body up, and because they can be moved easily.

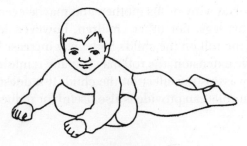

Figure 7.3
The lifting up of the child's body breaks up the abnormal pattern and gives her the experience
of a more normal posture. The movement of the roll can further reduce spasticity and
the child can be facilitated to carry out active movements in this new position

It is important to use the right size of roll for each child. If the roll is too small the child may not be lifted up high enough and not experience a useful new posture. If it is too big the child may be lifted too high for him to be able to be active.

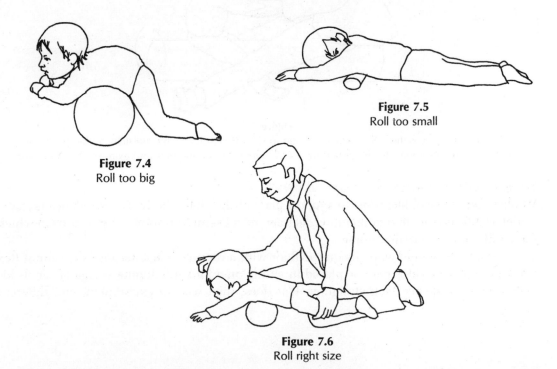

Figure 7.4
Roll too big

Figure 7.5
Roll too small

Figure 7.6
Roll right size

It is always necessary to check that the roll is doing the job you want. For example, if you want to help a child to actively extend his head and trunk in prone, you might place him over a roll so that his upper trunk is supported and he can take some weight on his forearms. For some children this will work well, and your treatment will succeed in getting him to actively lift his head to look at a toy or his mother, and maybe even reach forward with one hand as you work with his legs. For other children, however, it may have the opposite effect. The stimulation of the roll on the child's body may increase the flexor spasticity and, instead of facilitating active extension, the roll may actually reinforce the abnormal postural tone. You must constantly assess the effect on the child. If it doesn't work, don't do it.

The mobile support that rolls can provide is also useful for reducing spasticity in children with stiff pelvises.

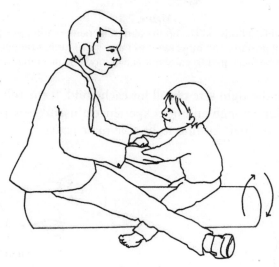

Figure 7.7
The therapist moves the roll slightly from side to side. This reduces the spasticity in the pelvis and allows active extension and rotation in the trunk with flexion at the hips and extension in the knees

Wedges (plastic-covered firm foam rubber)
Wedges can be used, like rolls, to support parts of the child's body. The difference is that a wedge is not mobile. In treatment, wedges are most useful in testing out positions in which the child may be placed at home.

For example, a child who sits on the floor with a rounded back because she cannot flex well enough at her hips may be placed in sitting on a forward-sloping wedge to see if this helps her to keep her back straighter. If it does, then we can experiment with different angles to see what works best. When we know the angle that works best, we can design a chair or floor cushion for the child that incorporates this angle. Other uses for wedges at home will be described later in this chapter.

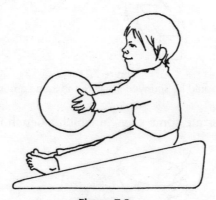

Figure 7.8
Using a wedge to reduce the amount of flexion in the hips
and facilitate long sitting with a straight back

Benches and stools

Strong, fairly heavy wooden stools and benches are essential for giving children the experience of sitting, and of changing position from the floor to sitting and from sitting to standing. Every centre should have a good selection of these so that it is possible to place children of all ages in sitting with their feet flat on the floor. Some of the taller stools can be used as tables to find the best height for arm support for a child who is sitting, or to give the child the possibility of using his hands.

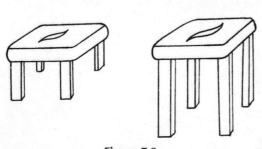

Figure 7.9
Stools varying in height from 10 cm to 60 cm—
some rectangular and some square

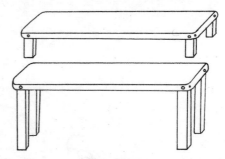

Figure 7.10
Benches varying in height from 15 cm to
30 cm and about 1 metre in length

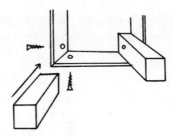

Figure 7.11
Legs should be screwed firmly to the frame around seat

The following pictures illustrate some ways in which a bench is useful.

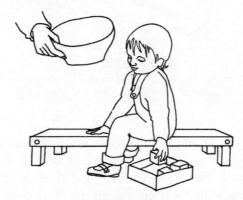

Figure 7.12
The child sits astride the bench so that active extension and rotation in his trunk can be facilitated while the adduction and internal rotation of his hips are reduced

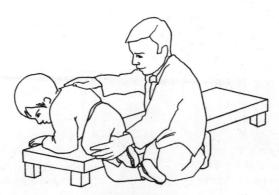

Figure 7.13
The child climbs onto and off the bench while the therapist facilitates rotation in his trunk

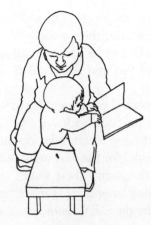

Figure 7.14
The child is supported in 'sandwich sitting',
where the therapist uses one leg to support
the child's pelvis from the back and another over
the child's legs to maintain the hips in a good
position, while the child is active in balancing
his trunk and head over this good base

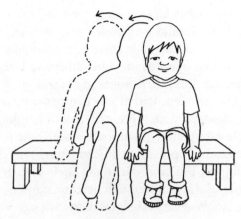

Figure 7.15
The bench is useful for a child to move
himself sideways in sitting

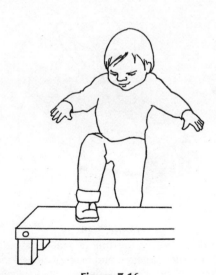

Figure 7.16
The bench is useful for a child to step on or off

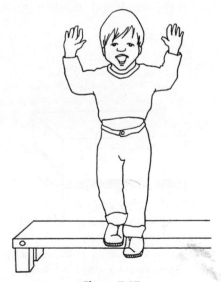

Figure 7.17
The bench is useful for a child to jump off

Standing tables

There are electrically operated tables that can change height at the touch of a switch, but if
these are not available an equally effective solution is to have a carpenter make a square

wooden table large enough for one or two children to sit at each side. The top and sides of the table should be covered first by a thin layer of sponge, and then a washable material. Each side of the table should accommodate children of different heights. On all sides there should be openings for the children's feet to pass through, so that the padded side of the table can hold their knees in extension.

The problem is that you can never have just little foot-sized openings that will be right for children with a great variety of heights. So it is more practical to leave one side of the table completely open for a wheelchair to go under, and have rectangular openings from the ground upwards at different heights in the other three sides for the various-sized standing children. But in order to get their feet through the openings and their knees supported, some of the children will need to stand on stools of various heights. It is more practical to use stools of varied heights than to design a table to accommodate all possible sizes, especially if the space in a treatment centre or school is limited.

The biggest children will have their feet flat on the floor. The smaller children will stand on stools and the openings in the side of the table will be higher up. The aim is to place the children in a semi-supported standing position so that their feet, hips and head are in alignment. The therapist will most likely need to use the pelvis as a key point of control to reduce flexion in the hips and facilitate the children's active extension, or to give them stability in the trunk and shoulder girdle.

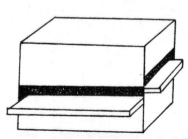

Figure 7.18
Table designed for children of different heights
to be supported in standing

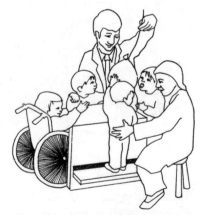

Figure 7.19
Children standing together at a table have the
opportunity to interact and play together during
therapy. This is also an opportunity for their
mothers to participate in therapy and learn
from the therapist and other mothers

Walking aids

Most centres have parallel bars. But these, in the way that they encourage the children to grasp and hang on with their hands, may not facilitate active mobile weight-bearing and balance reactions in the legs and trunk. It is worth trying to replace the normal hand rail with a flat plank so that, instead of grasping and pulling with his arms, the child can be facilitated to take weight on open hands and extended arms. Before he starts taking steps forwards, he should learn to take steps sideways inside the bars. Later, when he can balance with one foot in front of the other, he can learn to shift his weight from foot to foot. In children with spasticity, this weight shift will reduce the spasticity as long as the child is not fearful. Athetoid and ataxic children will benefit from the weight-bearing on both arms and legs, and also from experiencing the feeling of being upright and beginning to have some coordinated co-contraction in the trunk.

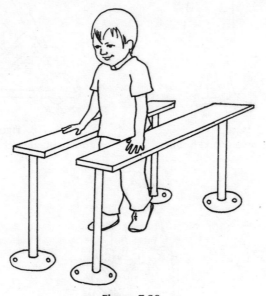

Figure 7.20
Parallel bars with flat board instead of handrail

In addition to parallel bars, there should be walking aids to try with children who are beginning to be able to take steps. These should only be of the kind that the family is allowed take home. It is cruel to have an expensive walking aid, kept only in the centre where the child can use it maybe for 10 minutes once a week, while at home he can only get about by crawling or holding on to the furniture.

Some children, particularly those with athetoid or ataxic CP, learn to walk by pushing a fairly heavy object, a chair or small table, in front of them. Holding on to the chair gives them symmetry and a steady point from which to move their legs. But children with spasticity need walking aids that facilitate hip extension. Walkers that the child pushes in front are more likely to facilitate hip flexion, and they will not enable him to develop balance reactions and eventually walk alone. Walkers that support the child from the back, and have a ratchet on the wheels to prevent them from being pushed backwards, *do* facilitate hip extension. Every effort should be made to develop cheap, local versions of this aid for those children who can take steps in them without their spasticity increasing.

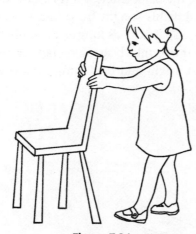

Figure 7.21
Pushing a chair gives symmetry and fixation

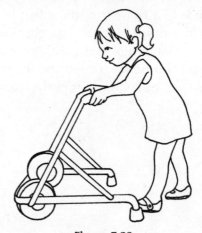

Figure 7.22
Rollator encourages child to walk with flexed hips

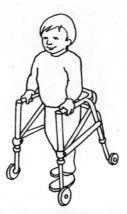

Figure 7.23
Back support walker facilitates extension of hips

Equipment to try out
Every centre should have a selection of chairs, standing frames and walking aids available for trying out. This way, the best piece of equipment can be found for children to use at home. It takes time for a child to become used to a new position and, before sending new equipment home with a child, the therapist must be sure that the child is safe in it and that

it does the job it has been designed for. For some children, the therapist may need several sessions to decide on the right piece of equipment and to test the child in it.

Splints
Sometimes, it is helpful to use light splints to keep a child's limb in extension to free your hands to work on another part of his body. For example, if you are working with a child with low tone in standing, you can free your hands to help him reach by putting gaiter splints on his legs to keep his knees in extension. These can be made of fabric with lightweight metal strips incorporated to hold them straight or, in a very young child, a few layers of newspaper fastened with sticky tape will be just enough to stop him from collapsing.

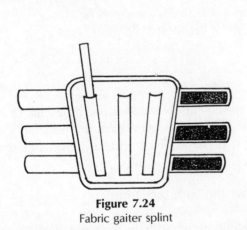

Figure 7.24
Fabric gaiter splint

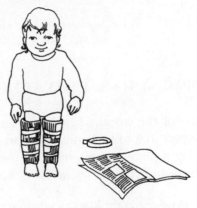

Figure 7.25
Newspaper and sellotape splint

Toys
The right kind of toys in a therapy department has a good impact on children and their families when they first attend. Seeing other children actively playing during therapy motivates both the child and his family to be actively involved. A broken doll and a therapist desperately snapping his fingers to attract a child's attention are very poor substitutes.

It is very important to keep the toys in a cupboard and take out only what is needed for a particular child at a particular time. Too many toys at once can be distracting and counter-productive. Having the right containers for the toys is also important, so that all the toys do not end up in a jumble of mixed pieces. Jigsaw puzzles need to be kept separate, with all their pieces intact. A set of blocks should be kept in one container, a set of objects specially collected for texture in another. Toys that are broken or incomplete should be repaired or thrown away.

In Appendix B, there is a table of possible play activities during therapy for children at different stages of development.

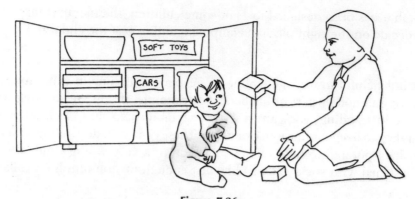

Figure 7.26
A tidy, well-arranged toy cupboard shows that therapists understand the
need for children to play, and the value of using play in therapy

EQUIPMENT TO BE USED AT HOME

In parts of the world where there are few therapists, children may have little chance of taking part in a full rehabilitation programme. They may, however, have the possibility of receiving a piece of equipment to use at home. It is therefore of crucial importance that therapists and community workers know how to:

- choose the right kind of equipment in partnership with the family,
- make sure the equipment fits the child well,
- explain to the family the way in which the equipment will help the child, and
- make sure the family know how to prepare the child before placing her in the equipment, how long she should spend in it and how active she should be.

Equipment that will be used by a child at home must be very carefully chosen. It is important to consider not just how it may or may not help the child, but also how it will be received by the family. Will they see it as something that is helpful to them in the way they care for the child? Is there room enough for it in the house? Will it be very difficult for them to position the child in it? Time needs to be taken to discuss these issues with the family. If a mother has asked for a chair so that she doesn't always have to make her child sit in her lap in order to feed her, then she will be more likely to use the chair when she gets it. If a therapist decides (for the best possible reasons) that a child needs a standing frame, but he hasn't taken time to discuss the situation with the family and explain why it may help their child, then he must not blame the family if they decide not to use it.

It has been observed that families who have opportunities to learn how to make their own equipment use that equipment with pride and confidence. Of course, not everyone can have this opportunity, but if the family are given the chance to share in the decision about what kind of equipment is best and how it should look, they will have a sense of ownership of it. They will value it more than if it just handed over to them because the therapist thinks it is a good idea.

One of the most difficult tasks is deciding which piece of equipment will be the most useful. Most families will ask for a chair, because it is easy to imagine how they and the child will benefit from the child being in a safe, comfortable sitting position. The trouble with sitting, however, is that it can fix the child in quite a lot of flexion, and it gives no opportunity for weight-bearing on the legs. In addition, it can be difficult, without complicated adaptations to the chair, to use the sitting position to give the child all he needs. On the one hand, he needs to learn to balance his trunk on his pelvis, to be symmetrical and to have a good base from which to use his hands. On the other, his mother needs him to be in a position in which she can easily feed him and also leave him for some times, knowing that he is safe and comfortable, while she gets on with other work.

A standing frame may be able to give the child all of these things more easily than a chair. It is more likely that he will be symmetrical in it, bear weight on his legs, have good opportunities to balance his trunk on his pelvis and, if he has a table in front, use his hands. For many children, even eating and drinking can be easier in a standing frame than in a chair. Most important, the majority of children are happier to be in standing, at least for short periods.

But this is a strange idea for many families and it may take time and sensitive persuasion before they can accept it. It may be necessary to give them a chair at home at first, and to demonstrate at the centre over a number of weeks how the standing frame may be better. If they live in a very small house and have room for only one piece of equipment, they will need to be totally convinced of the benefit of the standing frame before they will be ready to give up the chair. Of course, most children will benefit from having both a chair and a standing frame.

Every piece of equipment must be safe for the child to use. It must be carefully explained to the family that a child must not be left for too long (usually not more than half an hour) in any position, and that he should not be left alone, particularly in standing frames.

The following are some pieces of equipment that might be useful for families to have at home.

Wedges

These are useful for positioning a child for short periods. Those children who are able to lift their heads a little when placed in prone over a wedge may benefit from this, as long as they are left with toys within reach. The family must be sure, however, that the child will not roll over and fall off. If there is any danger of this, sandbags should be placed on either side of the child.

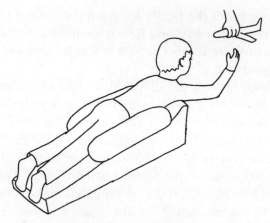

Figure 7.27
Prone over wedge supported with sandbags

Children in danger of hip dislocation because of the adduction and internal rotation of their hips when they are left lying supine, may benefit from having their legs flexed over a wedge. This breaks up the pattern of spasticity and also gives them symmetry.

Children who push back into extension when they lie on their backs may benefit from having their nappies changed while lying on a low wedge. The wedge should flex their hips just enough to reduce the spasticity.

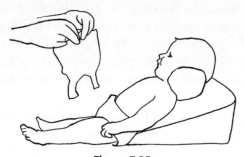

Figure 7.28
Wedge giving hip flexion to prevent push back into extension.
Neck cushion elongates neck and prevents extension

Side-lying board

This is useful for children who are very floppy, and for those children who push back into extension when they are left supine but who cannot tolerate being left in prone.

The board can be made of cardboard or wood. If it is made of wood, it should be covered in a thin layer of sponge and washable fabric. The front support should be high enough to prevent the child from rolling over into supine, but small enough to allow free movement of her arms. It should be in the middle of the board so that sometimes the child can be placed on her right side and sometimes on her left. She should always have a small firm pillow under her head.

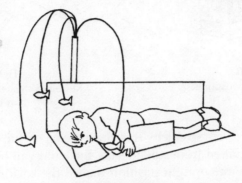

Figure 7.29
The side-lying position gives children symmetry and allows them to bring their hands together in front of their eyes. It is helpful to have some toys suspended near their hands

Chairs (special seating)
In countries with adequate resources, chairs which can be adapted to all kinds of children are often available. They can be changed to allow the child to relax in them or to be active in them. They 'grow' with the child, and they can easily be moved around. Even so, because they are so expensive, it is not easy for every child to have the right chair exactly when it is needed. In this book we only have space to describe chairs that are simple in design and easily reproduced.

The following are descriptions of a selection of chairs that can be made using appropriate paper-based technology (APT) or wood. For each one, there are suggestions as to which children may benefit from them and why. The design for making a basic chair with APT, and the way of taking measurements, will be found in Appendix A.

1. Reclining chair
This is modelled on the small chair used for normal babies. It supports the child in a re-clining position, upright enough so that she can see what is going on around her but not so upright that she is in any danger of flexing forwards.

This chair is useful for a child with very low tone. It gives him the possibility of being a little upright and, if a table is placed in front of him at chest height, of perhaps being able to use his hands. A neck pillow may be needed to help keep the child's head in midline, and a foot-board will help to give support to his feet.

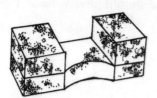

Figure 7.30
Neck cushion made of sponge

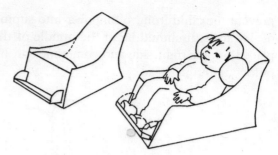

Figure 7.31
Reclining chair showing neck cushion
and foot-board

For an older child with severe spasticity this chair is also useful, especially for feeding. If the chair back is slightly curved from side to side, the child will be more comfortable and may be able to tolerate a more upright position than if the back is flat. It is important to make sure that the child's pelvis is right back in the seat. Groin straps may be needed to keep the pelvis back, and also to keep the hips outwardly rotated. A padded post between his legs will not work as well, because the child is likely to push against it using abnormal extension, and this will increase his adductor spasticity.

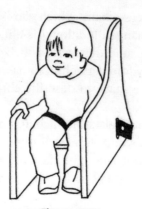

Figure 7.32
Groin straps must be fastened at the right angle to outwardly rotate the hips

2. Upright chair and table

Children who have some head and trunk control should be placed in upright chairs rather than reclining chairs. This is because they need the experience of being upright so that they can begin to hold the position for themselves. If a child has quite low tone and falls forward, or if there is some pulling down into the flexion pattern in his arms, the table should be at chest height.

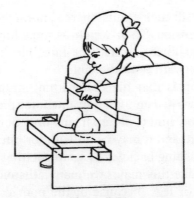

Figure 7.33
Upright chair showing support at chest height and knee blocks

This kind of chair is useful for children with moderate spastic quadriplegia. Make sure that his pelvis is not pulled back more on one side than on the other, and that he is not sitting back on his sacrum. It may be necessary to use knee blocks to push his pelvis to the back of the seat and to hold his hips in some abduction. This will give him a good base from which to be able to use his hands.

3. Prone angle (forward-tilting) chair

Children with poor trunk control who go into total extension pattern when they lift their heads have great difficulty sitting in an upright chair. As soon as they lift their heads, their arms lift up into abduction and outward rotation and they cannot bring them forward onto the table. These children need to be in a forward-tipped sitting position supported at chest height from the front.

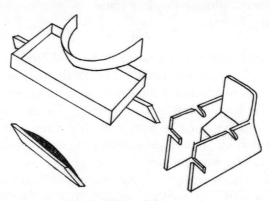

Figure 7.34
The forward-tipped position reduces extensor spasticity

In this position, when they lift their heads, there is nothing to push against and they are not likely to go into total extension. Their weight is tipped forward by the sloping seat so that they take weight on their knees against the knee blocks and on the chest support. Their hands can then come forward onto the table.

The benefit of this position is that the child is not strapped tightly in to the chair. The curved chest support allows just enough movement for the child to learn some postural control, but not enough to allow him to slump in any direction. The angle of the seat of the chair is critical. Too far forward and it may be difficult for him to lift his head at all, too far back and he is in danger of pushing backwards again. Getting it right needs a lot of experimenting, but having a chair like this may save many athetoid children from trying to fix themselves using their arms or legs, because of the poor co-contraction in their trunk. Without such a chair, an athetoid child can develop strong flexor spasticity in his arms and legs, and these can lead to painful contractures and deformities later in life.

Standing frames

All through this book there has been a strong emphasis on the need to give children with CP opportunities to take weight on their legs. Being in a standing position can give a child a greater possibility of symmetry, learning postural control, avoiding contractures and deformities, and being in a position that is enjoyable and satisfying. It is not possible for family members to hold a child in a good standing position for more than 5–10 minutes at a time. This is not long enough for the child to benefit much. He may need half an hour two or three times a day, depending on how much he enjoys it and also on how necessary it may be to prevent him from getting into more harmful positions such as W-sitting or crawling.

There are two main kinds of standing frame that are useful for children with CP:

1. A prone angle (forward-tilting) standing frame.
2. An upright standing frame.

In some centres, standing frames which support the child from behind (supine standers) are used. In these, the child leans backwards in the standing position. *These are not recommended.* The reason is, first of all, that it does not feel at all normal for the child. Second, and more important, in order to reach forward with her hands and to look at what she is doing, she must actively *flex* in her hips and trunk. Children with CP who are trying to learn to stand need to develop active hip *extension* against gravity. So, supine standing frames actually encourage the wrong action.

Prone angle standing frames, on the other hand, tip the child forward slightly so that every time he lifts his head and trunk and uses his hands he may be facilitated to actively extend his hips. This does, however, very much depend on the standing frame supporting him in just the right way. The points to check carefully are:

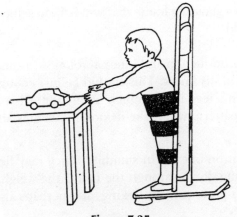

Figure 7.35
Supine standing frame

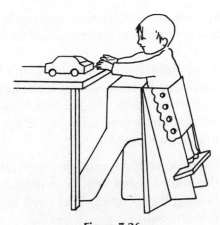

Figure 7.36
Prone angle standing frame

1. Does the pelvic belt hold the hips in extension so that the child's head, hips and heels are in alignment? This will depend on the side supports being just the right width. If they are too wide, the child's hips will flex inside the belt and there will be no possibility of active hip extension. If they are too narrow, the belt will hold the child too tightly and he will just hang on the belt, and again there will be no active hip extension.

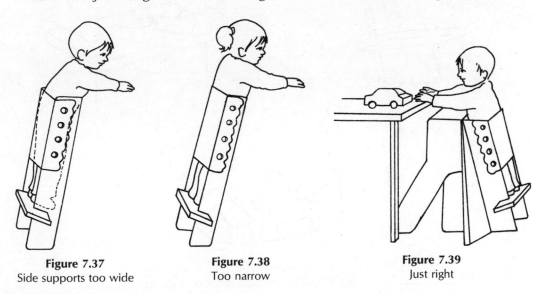

Figure 7.37
Side supports too wide

Figure 7.38
Too narrow

Figure 7.39
Just right

2. Is the angle of the frame upright enough so that he can actively extend his head and trunk, but not so upright that he has no need to actively extend?

There are many adaptations that can be made to a standing frame that will help to achieve the best position and active movement in the child.

- If the child stands in the frame with his legs in adduction and internal rotation, a small block can be built into the frame at the level of his knees. This should be just enough to prevent adduction but should not place his legs in too much abduction. This is because abduction, being part of the flexion pattern, will make flexion in his hips and knees more likely.

- Athetoid children very often only take weight on one leg in standing. They may flex the other leg and then be in danger of slipping down through the belt if the weight-bearing leg collapses. They need heel cups to prevent them flexing, and perhaps also foot-straps to keep both feet flat.

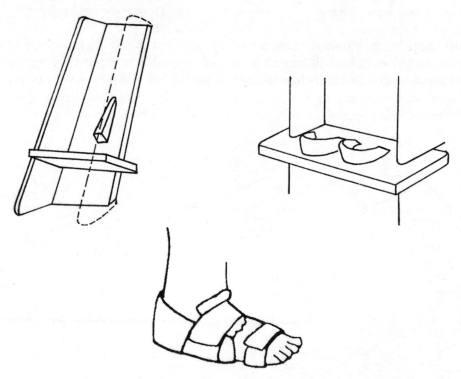

Figure 7.40
Abduction block, heel cups and foot-straps

- Dystonic children may suddenly push back into extension when standing in the frame. They may even push the whole frame over backwards. To prevent this, an extension can be made to the pelvic belt, with long straps around the shoulders that fasten to the table in front. This will keep the shoulder girdle protracted (pulled forwards) and prevent a full extensor thrust.

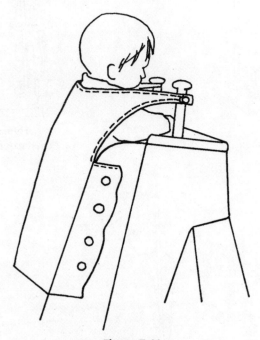

Figure 7.41
Straps to keep shoulder girdle from pushing backwards

Standing frames can be made of APT or of wood. If they are made of wood, the front panel should be covered in sponge and washable material. This should not be too thick or soft, otherwise the child's knees will be able to flex into it.

Preparing the child

A great deal of care needs to be taken while putting a child into a standing frame. If she has spasticity this should first be reduced and then the child should be lifted into the frame without losing the good position. Some toys should be placed on the table beforehand so that, if she is apprehensive, she will have something to take her mind off her worries. The pelvic belt should be fastened first and the foot-straps and shoulder straps later, if they are needed. *Never* fasten the foot-straps first, in case the child should have a sudden extensor thrust and fall out. If this were to happen and her feet were fixed, she would be very likely to have a fractured tibia or fibula in both legs.

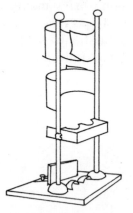

Figure 7.42
Upright stander

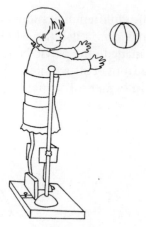

Figure 7.43
Active extension of hips

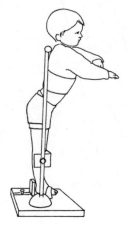

Figure 7.44
Extension of lumbar spine—no active extension in hips

Upright standing frames are useful for children who have good head and trunk control but cannot stand alone for long without using their hands for support. Being in the standing frame makes them accustomed to not relying on their hands.

Care should be taken, however, in deciding on an upright standing frame. Remember that in order for a child to be able to stand alone, he needs good active extension in his hips and knees. If he is not getting opportunities to actively extend his hips and knees in the upright stander, then he is not getting good preparation for standing alone. Some children may hang on the belts of the stander and actively extend only in the lumbar spine. Check this is not the case before you decide.

An upright standing frame can be made of wood or metal with wide straps and velcro fastening to support the pelvis and chest. The knees are supported by curved, padded wooden blocks just below the knee joint. The feet are held by heel cups and straps.

Inserts

In wheelchairs and pushchairs, children need to be given good sitting positions so that they will be comfortable and so that they can use the opportunity to develop better postural control.

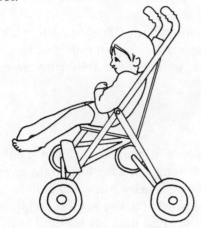

Figure 7.45
Poor sitting position in pushchair

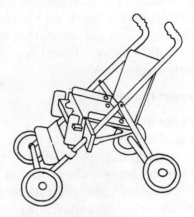

Figure 7.46
Insert attached to pushchair

Rather than making complicated systems of straps that family members may find tiresome to fasten, APT inserts may hold the child in a good position. For example, a child who sits back on his sacrum and has windswept hips in sitting could have an insert with knee blocks in his wheelchair. A child who pushes back into extension could have a prone angle insert with chest support in her pushchair.

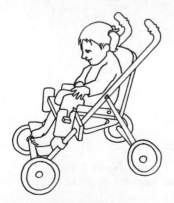

Figure 7.47
Improved sitting position of child

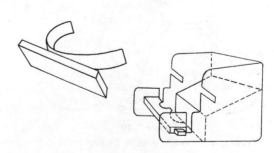

Figure 7.48
Prone angle insert for pushchair

Ride-on walkers

Children who move around on the floor, either in crawling with too much flexion, or by pushing themselves along on their backs, are in danger of contractures and deformities and also of not developing good function either in their arms and hands or in their legs. Developing alternative means of moving around is necessary.

Let me first of all say that baby walkers are not acceptable. This is because they support the child in such a way that he can use his spasticity to push himself about or, if he has athetoid or ataxic CP, he is given no opportunity to develop postural control and uses asymmetrical movements to get about. Also, most children with CP learning to walk are taller than the 1-year-old babies that walkers are designed for. This means that they will therefore walk with very flexed legs if they use such walkers. The following are more appropriate suggestions.

Tricycle with the pedals cut off

Wooden horse

This is a useful aid for a child who has good enough balance to sit alone. The seat should be high enough off the ground to allow her to push herself along using her feet on the ground, without her legs being too bent. At first she will push herself backwards using both feet but later, with some help, she will learn to go forwards and perhaps to use her feet reciprocally. Take care not to choose a tricycle with a very wide seat because then her legs will be in too much abduction and it will be hard for her to extend them.

For older children, it may be possible to use a bicycle with trainer wheels, and for children whose sitting balance is not reliable, it may be possible to attach a trunk support ring to the tricycle.

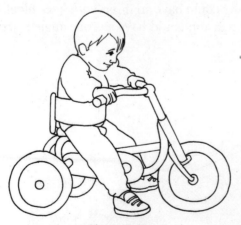

Figure 7.49
Using legs on the floor to propel tricycle

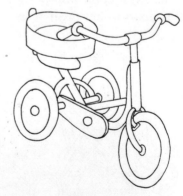

Figure 7.50
Trunk support ring attached to tricycle

This horse has four castors that can move freely in any direction and is easy to make. The seat is narrow and can be covered with a firm cushion shaped to keep the child's legs in some abduction and outward rotation. The seat and handles can be moved up as the child grows. The wooden horse will be useful for a child who has good sitting balance.

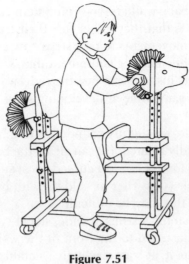

Figure 7.51
Wooden horse

APT wheeled walkers

It is difficult to find suitable walkers for athetoid children, particularly those with dystonic spasms. Since the main problem with many athetoid children is that they do not have adequate co-contraction and stability in the trunk, they tend to compensate for this by fixing the upper parts of their body in extreme positions in order to move their legs. I have seen

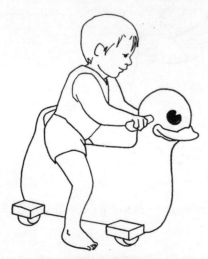

Figure 7.52
Walker with no trunk support

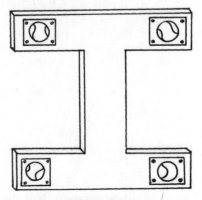

Figure 7.53
The base of this walker is wood. It is fitted with four castors so that it can move in any direction

children in homemade large baby walker–type equipment careering around a room having such good fun. The problem is that they either flex their trunk forward or push back into extension and then use head movements to take steps. Since it is so important for a child to be able to move, it is worthwhile making equipment that will help him to do this in a good way. The APT walker supports his trunk in just the right way, so that he can learn to move his legs and take steps at the same time as developing some coordinated co-contraction in his trunk.

The walker has a rather narrow, slightly rounded sitting base, so that the child's legs are slightly abducted and outwardly rotated. He can sit on the base itself, or a more supportive saddle can be made. He leans forward onto a curved chest support, with a fairly broad strap fastened with velcro across his back. He can hold on with his hands if this is possible, but with many athetoid children this may be difficult.

If her arms have strong dystonic spasms, a wide, shawl-type band can be placed around her shoulders and arms and fastened to the front of the walker. This may seem rather restrictive but, if she can tolerate it, at least it will give a child with these difficult spasms the possibility of using her fairly good legs for weight-bearing, moving around and having fun.

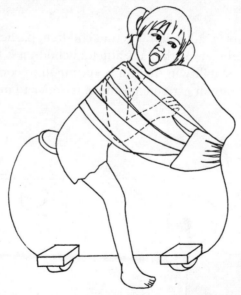

Figure 7.54
Use of shoulder straps to prevent dystonic spasms and give child a fixed base from which to move

Toilet chairs

Teaching a child to be clean and dry is one of the most important things for any family. Children with CP may have extra difficulties with learning this because of the problems they have with maintaining positions. They may be fearful when placed on a toilet or pot, because their balance is unreliable or because they cannot sit comfortably.

Normally, a child will squat to pass urine or faeces. This position is the most effective one for using the abdominal muscles to empty the bowel. But for children with CP, squatting is very difficult because it is such a flexed position. In order to balance, they need to be lifted up off the ground a little. This can be done on a child's pot which has a wide base, or the child can have a special chair made from wood or APT with a plastic covering on the seat.

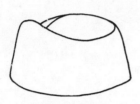

Figure 7.55
Steady, wide-based pot

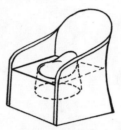

Figure 7.56
Toliet chair

When the child is first learning to use the toilet or a pot, he will need to be held securely by his mother so that he can feel safe. Once he has learnt how to pass urine or faeces in the pot and he is confident about it, then he can start learning to balance more on his own. If he has some sitting balance but needs to hold on with his hands, the pot can be placed inside a cardboard box which has a bar across it that he can hold. The sides of the box and the bar to hold will give him security.

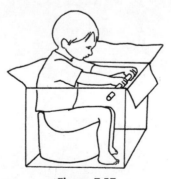

Figure 7.57
Pot inside cardboard box

If, however, he is the kind of child who pushes back all the time, he may need to be supported from the front. If he already has a forward-tilting chair, perhaps this could be adapted to double as a toilet chair. A hole could be cut in the seat and the remaining surface covered in strong, washable plastic. A flat board could be placed over the hole when he uses the chair other than in the toilet.

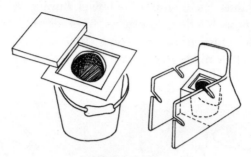

Figure 7.58
Adapted forward-tilting chair

Bathing aids

Most children enjoy the experience of being bathed. This is true, however, only if they feel safe. When the child is fairly small and if he has some sitting balance, he will feel safe in a bathtub as long as someone is close by. If he is the kind of child who sits back on his sacrum and whose upper back is rounded, he will be helped by sitting up on a semi-inflated swimming ring which is propped up at the back on a firm piece of sponge. If one ring does not help him enough, try two rings tied together.

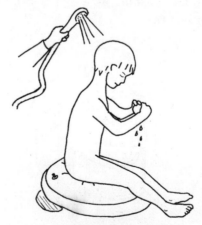

Figure 7.59
Sitting on a semi-inflated ring may give a child just enough support to help him learn to balance

Until a child has good sitting balance, it is helpful for him to have a towel to sit on. This gives him a less slippery surface on which to balance.

A child whose sitting balance is not so good will need some support while being bathed. If the mother is doing this alone, either she must hold onto the child with one hand and wash him with the other, or she will need a special support in which she can place him and know he will be safe.

It is important to help the family member who bathes the child to find a good position to be in so that they can hold the child safely but not damage their own backs. Kneeling on a soft cushion is usually better than stooping over. If kneeling is difficult, sitting on a low stool may be an alternative.

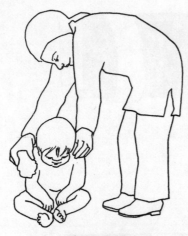

Figure 7.60
Stooping over the child is damaging for the mother's back

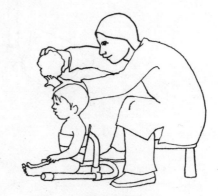

Figure 7.61
Sitting on a low stool is better

Cheap PVC plumbing pipes with connections can be bought in most places. They are very useful for making washable bath aids. The one in Figure 7.62 has a trunk support made

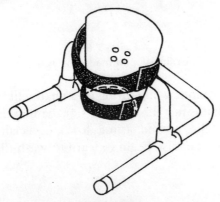

Figure 7.62
Supporting chair made of PVC pipes

from an empty plastic container and fixed to the pipes with cable ties. The straps are made of towelling and Velcro.

Shower aids

For bigger children, showering is easier than bathing. If the child has no sitting balance but does not push back too much into extension, then a chair made of plastic pipes (Figure 7.62) may give him the support he needs. If the child does push back into extension and cannot be made comfortable in such a chair, a side-lying support may be the answer.

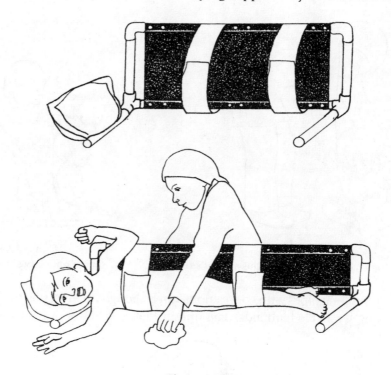

Figure 7.63
Side-lying support made of PVC pipes

Children who can balance alone while sitting on a chair will benefit from having a plastic chair with wide openings that is just the right size for them in the shower. They can use the opportunity to practise standing up and sitting down, especially if there is a firm handrail for them to hold on to. They can also begin to learn to wash themselves.

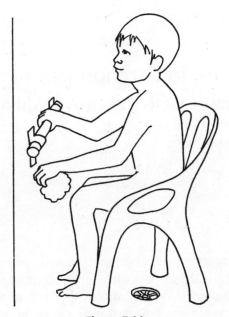

Figure 7.64
A light plastic chair that is the right height is good for a child to use in the shower

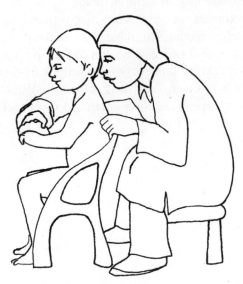

Figure 7.65
Hand-over-hand learning to wash herself

Chapter 8

Sensory integration problems in children with cerebral palsy

ANNIE BROZAITIS

WHAT IS SENSORY INTEGRATION?

ENSORY integration is a normal part of human life. Without it we would not be able to make contact with our surrounding world. Our senses allow us to see, hear, smell, taste and touch; they tell us the position of our muscles and joints, as well as our movement, direction and balance. Receptors in our bodies transmit this sensory information in a continual flow to our brains, where it is constantly being processed, so that an appropriate response can be made.

For instance, the receptors in your inner ears may transmit information to the brain that you are losing your balance, having stumbled. The brain processes this information and sends a message to the muscles needed to respond to keep your body upright.

Sensory information is received and processed in the sub-cortical (or lower brain stem) area, as shown in Figure 8.1. From there it is transmitted up to the cortical area, where sensori-motor control takes place, enabling organised movement.

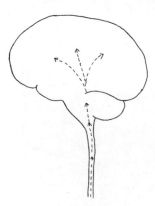

Figure 8.1

Cerebral palsy is caused by damage to the nervous system, specifically the cortical and sub-cortical areas of the brain. Although it is movement control and the sensation of movement that are mainly affected, a child with CP may also have lower brain stem sensory integration dysfunction—that is, the incoming sensory information is not being correctly processed. His restricted movements in themselves also interfere with normal sensory processing. He then has inaccurate information about his muscle activity, the position of his limbs and where his body is in space, which makes normal movement even more difficult for him. This difficulty in organising and integrating sensory information affects his ability to move, learn, explore his surroundings, pay attention and behave appropriately in a situation.[1]

Because he lacks the experience of purposeful movement, a child with CP also has less possibility of touching and grasping his own body, exploring his surroundings and manipulating objects and toys. His tactile development is affected. As a result, he may have poor development of body awareness, perception of touch and discrimination, and possibly may not be able to tolerate certain textures.

Thus, a child with sensory integration problems may have:

- Problems with movement coordination.
- Balance problems.
- Difficulty planning new movements.
- Slowness in adapting to different positions.
- Lack of awareness of where his body is in space.
- The inability to understand the nature of the objects or textures that he touches.

Knowing about these problems of sensory integration may help parents and carers of children with CP to understand some of their children's more subtle difficulties. For example, parents will often say that their child is fearful of sitting on the toilet, even when she is adequately supported. She may become upset or distressed when eating certain foods or touching soft toys, or seem unaware of certain parts of her body and how to use them, even though she moves and walks using a supportive frame. This chapter will explore how to assess what a child's sensory processing difficulties are, and will identify the principles involved in treating them.

The theory of sensory integration

Sensory integration, as a theory, was developed in the 1960s by the occupational therapist and psychologist Jean Ayres. She first became interested in sensory processing when treating children with delayed coordination and apparent learning difficulties. In the 1970s and 1980s, Ayres and others[2] began extending their theory to look at the sensory processing of

[1] Blanche 2000, DeGangi 1994, 2000.
[2] Moore 1984.

children with CP. In recent years, interest in this area has increased. It is now recognised that children with CP have sensory processing difficulties as well as motor deficits.[3] Increasingly, therapists are using their sensory integration knowledge to help understand and treat motor and functional difficulties in children with CP.[4]

Jean Ayres defined sensory integration as the ability of the central nervous system to receive, process and organise sensory stimulus, and to translate this into an adaptive response. This process is continuous, generally subconscious, and gives us ongoing information about our own bodies and the environment. Ayres placed particular importance in her theory on the following three 'proximal' senses.

Proprioception

This sense gives us constant information about the position of our joints and limbs, our movement and body position. Even when our eyes are closed, for instance, we know exactly where our hands, legs and arms are. Proprioception tells us if muscles are stretching or contracting and when and where limbs are bending and straightening. It has a major influence on our overall body awareness, movement planning and control. Receptors for the proprioceptive sense are located in the receptors of the muscles, joints, ligaments and tendons.

Vestibular

Receptors within our inner ears detect all the movements we make and tell us about changes in the position of our heads. Movement and gravity stimulate the vestibular receptors, influencing our body position, our perception of movement and whether we perceive objects as moving or still in relation to our body. It has been called the three-dimensional centre, as it gives us basic information about ourselves in relation to gravity and space. It is the vestibular system, for instance, that is affected by spinning and makes us feel dizzy. When it does not function effectively, the interpretation of our other senses is affected, becoming inaccurate and inconsistent.

Tactile

Sensory cells located within our skin receive and interpret information about touch, pain, temperature, pressure, vibration and movement. The tactile system interprets information that helps us to make sense of our surroundings. It plays a large part in our emotional stability and influences the functional skills we need for everyday activities. It also plays an important role in body awareness and our ability to focus our attention.

Sensory integration theory describes how the three proximal senses are processed and organised in the lower part of the brain stem and thalamus. This process begins even before

---

[3] Blanche 2000, Lesny et al. 1993.
[4] Blanche 2000, DeGangi 1994, 2000.

a child is born. The baby's experiences of movement, changes of position, temperature of the amniotic fluid, sounds and the feeling of having her thumb in her mouth are early sensations that help the development of her central nervous system. The development and integration of these proximal sensations continue to dominate early child development. They form a secure base on which the more complex skills such as detailed movement planning, regulated behaviour, attention, communication, learning and visual perception, among others, can be developed and refined.

HYPOSENSITIVITY AND HYPERSENSITIVITY

Everyone integrates sensory information differently. For example, some children dislike playgrounds and funfairs, or being touched and tickled, whereas others seem to crave these experiences and sensations. These are different sensory responses to the same sensory experiences.

Hyposensitivity — — — — — — — — — — — — **Hypersensitivity**

Most of us would fall within the middle range of the continuum, varying between under- (hypo-) and over- (hyper-) sensitivity. Our ability to take in, organise and respond to sensory information will alter from day to day, depending on how tired, hungry, anxious or overloaded we are. However, when the nervous system has a pronounced overreaction or under-reaction to incoming sensations, or fluctuates between the two, there is a difficulty of sensory processing. The child that intensely dislikes funfairs could be hypersensitive to sensory information, whereas the child who craves sensory experiences could be hyposensitive.

A child who is under- or hyposensitive will register sensory information less intensely and will not receive adequate information. For example, she may not notice being touched, she may like lots of movement or seem unaware of parts of her body. A hyposensitive child requires extra sensory activity to have better awareness and to help her maintain her arousal and attention. If this is not obtained through normal daily life or during treatment, she may start to 'seek out' the sensations her sensory system needs. For example, to gain better tactile and proprioceptive information, she may repeatedly bite hard on objects in her mouth.

A child who registers sensory information in an over- or hypersensitive way could be very irritable; he may dislike being touched or touching certain textures, or become quickly frightened by movement. He may 'avoid' the sensations that he is unable to tolerate. For example, he might become rigid and fixed in one position so as not to move, or dislike playing with and exploring soft and furry toys.

A child that fluctuates between hypo- and hypersensitivity can be very reactive to touch or movement at some times but not at others, sensitive to some things and not to others.

This is known as a sensory modulation difficulty, whereby the brain cannot easily adapt to and balance the incoming sensory information.

Children with these problems often struggle to carry out functional daily tasks even though their motor difficulties are not severe. Frequently they show problems in maintaining their level of arousal and attention.[5]

EXAMPLES OF SENSORY PROCESSING PROBLEMS IN CHILDREN WITH CP

Athetoid CP

A child with athetoid CP will often be hyposensitive. He enjoys repeated amounts of movement, usually in the form of swinging. He does not easily become dizzy and will tolerate much more activity than many children who have no disability. He tends to enjoy tactile and proprioceptive sensations: being touched firmly, being stroked with a body mitt, *deep pressure* to his joints, vibration, and weight on his limbs. The toys and objects he tends to enjoy are firm, giving clear tactile feedback.

Spasticity

In contrast, a child with spasticity can show signs of hypersensitivity. She can be quite fearful of movement, becoming rigid and distressed; her tone can increase even with the slightest sensation of motion. This may be due to lack of postural control and delayed saving reactions, combined with the sensory processing problem of 'gravitational insecurity'. Gravitional insecurity is primarily a vestibular processing problem which makes a child feel highly anxious that she will fall when her head and body position changes.

Children with spasticity also frequently have:

- poor body awareness,
- problems with motor planning (movement organisation), and
- difficulty with bilateral integration, which is using two hands together in a coordinated manner.

[5] For more detail on sensory integration theroy, see DeGangi 1994, Blanche et al. 1995, Fisher et al. 1991, Stock Kranowitz 1998 and Roley et al. 2001.

These are out of proportion to the movement restrictions they experience due to abnormal postural tone.

Besides this, children with spasticity have unusual sensitivity to tactile sensations. They may be either hypersensitive (for example, unable to tolerate furry, soft or messy textures) or they may seem under-responsive or hyposensitive to tactile sensations (unable to locate where they have been touched, unaware of their clothing or not noticing food around their mouths, for instance).

Pre-term children

New information from clinical studies about children born pre-term, or of extremely low birth weight, describes sensory processing difficulties, and also problems with self-regulation.[6] Children with a self-regulation difficulty struggle to establish a sleep/wake cycle, or to gain a regular pattern of feeding. They are also unable to easily calm and settle themselves or to control their emotional responses. Children that are born pre-term and who have CP frequently have sensory processing difficulties. They can initially show some hypersensitivity to movement, needing careful support and positioning. They usually find it easier to settle when 'nested' (wrapped closely in a cloth), or swaddled, as the consistent tactile and proprioceptive input helps them to feel safe and comfortable. They can then become calm with rhythmical gentle rocking. These children are also very often hypersensitive to tactile sensations.

Other causes

Other children with CP who often have sensory processing difficulties are those who are cared for within an institution, or where no therapy has been available to them or their families. These children have often missed out on important early physical contact, and are frequently left in one position, without experience of movement or changes in body position. It may be difficult to give them the consistent daily care of feeding, washing and dressing that they need. Clinical experience of working with children in these situations shows that their emotional and sensory development has been affected.

Recently, interest and research into the area of 'emotional attachment and security and sensory processing' has increased. It is now acknowledged that there is a close link between emotional care and stability and sensory processing problems (as Eadaoin Bhreathnach's work shows). For this reason, and of course those already mentioned, children with CP who do not have parents or regular carers to look after them need a sensitive and consistent approach.

[6] DeGangi 1994, 2000, Anderson 1996.

HOW CAN WE ASSESS A CHILD'S SENSORY INTEGRATION PROBLEMS?

Gathering information about the child's sensory processing can be done by careful observation and discussion with parents, carers, other therapists, nursery staff and teachers. The observation should be done in a variety of settings, for example, at home, in a play area, at school or during therapy sessions.

General observations

Observe carefully how the child responds to the sensations of movement, touch or a play activity. How are his movement patterns, postural tone, body temperature, mouthing reactions and facial expressions affected? For instance, he may appear distressed: his postural tone may increase, his breathing may change or he may become fidgety and start pulling faces. (In this case always stop and change the activity.)

Take notice of how a child organises or plans his movements. Does he become stuck in one position? He may have sufficient postural tone and movement control to carry out a variety of sequenced movements, but be unable to do so. If this is the case, it is likely to be due to a sensory processing difficulty affecting the child's ability to initiate, plan, organise and perform varied, directional and sequenced movements.

The following observations can help us to determine whether or not there is a sensory integration difficulty:

- What activity does the child choose or avoid?
- What toys does he prefer or dislike?
- Can he plan how to move on, off, through, under or over objects?
- Can he organise himself when asked to copy or carry out actions?
- How does he respond to being moved, for example, sitting with minimal support on a bench, or sitting on a slightly moving surface such as a ball, roll, tricycle or swing?
- Is he having difficulty developing the skills of handwriting, drawing and cutting?
- Can he concentrate, or is he easily distracted?
- During washing, dressing, eating and drinking, does he have a difficulty that is not explained by abnormal tone?

If a child does not respond typically to input which is normally effective for his or her movement disorder, it is worth assuming that there may be a sensory processing problem.

Specific observations

If the child does seem to have a sensory processing dysfunction, the following table will help us to gather information in different surroundings (such as from family, carers and teachers) to make a more specific assessment.

Specific observations to assess sensory integration problems (1)

Hypersensitivity		
Tactile	Vestibular	Proprioceptive
• Dislikes dressing and undressing or likes to be clothed • Feels uncomfortable with certain textures of clothing; overly aware of labels and waistbands • Becomes irritable when having hair brushed, nails cut or teeth cleaned • Avoids touching textures such as grass, sand, finger paints, play dough, furry toys. Dislikes having messy hands • Too much tactile stimulation causes increased mouthing, tongue movement, drooling or vomiting; or increased breathing rate, perspiration or fidgeting • Touches toys and other tools with the tips of fingers • Prefers certain food textures: only hard and crunchy, or only soft • Dislikes people being too close; is uncomfortable being cuddled or held • Calms down with deep pressure, firm touch or when wrapped/swaddled tightly • Has difficulty maintaining a grasp to hold and manipulate toys and objects (over and above problems with movement control and postural tone) • Has poor concentration and attention	• Is quickly affected/upset by sudden movement • Easily suffers motion sickness • Can look fearful—e.g., with rapidly increased postural tone and hands tightly fisted—at being moved suddenly • Dislikes having feet unsupported • Dislikes swinging and playground activities • Avoids changes of direction and position • Can be slow in moving onto a chair, bench or off the floor • Dislikes moving backwards even if well supported • Objects to sitting on a therapy ball • Is slow to learn to walk, go up and down stairs or ride a tricycle (relevant for children with mild CP)	• This difficulty is far less common and quite difficult to detect; however, it can occur. A child may become uncomfortable and distressed when placed in positions where she is weight-bearing. She is also unable to tolerate her joints being moved passively. This defensiveness to proprioceptive input 'can be part of an overall sensory defensiveness pattern' (Blanche 2000)

Specific observations to assess sensory integration problems (2)

	Hyposensitivity	
Tactile	Vestibular	Proprioceptive
• May not notice being touched	• Enjoys movement activities, e.g., on a swing or therapy ball	• Looks for support, and likes to feel deep pressure
• Enjoys being handled, seeks out cuddles and contact	• Can tolerate greater amounts of very active movement than would be expected, e.g., spinning, swinging and bouncing	• Responds to compression and tapping techniques
• Seems not to notice pain, e.g., scratches, bruises		• Likes firm toys to play with, and enjoys banging and pushing
• Bites or hits self		• Bites on objects, likes hard, crunchy foods and often chews clothing
• Seems unaware when messy around mouth or nose	• Does not become dizzy when other children would	
• Does not notice when clothes are twisted	• Seeks out opportunities for movement	• Does not easily adapt his body posture to changes of position
• Explores objects with her mouth	• Has poor increase of extensor tone with linear movements, i.e., forwards and backwards	• May have low proximal tone
• Likes vibration, often on hands and around the mouth		• Poor body awareness and lack of trunk rotation
• Tactile discrimination difficulty (age 2 and above)	• Likes to be upside-down during play	• Has problems with motor planning and sequencing activities
• Has fine motor difficulties above the effect of any abnormal postural tone, e.g., doing and undoing buttons, holding a pencil, or using scissors		• May over-fill mouth and lose food when eating
		• Has difficulty maintaining grasp and struggles to manipulate pencils, scissors and buttons, over and above difficulties due to abnormal postural tone
• Needs to look at hands when carrying out activities		• Looks for support, and likes to feel deep pressure
• Frequently explores an object by putting it in her mouth		• Responds to compression and tapping techniques

PRINCIPLES OF TREATMENT

As no two children with CP are the same, so no two treatment programmes will be identical, but will be based on observations of the child's needs. With every child, the treatment aims to give exactly the right level of sensory input, so that the information can be processed and integrated in a more balanced and regular way.

Under the headings of the three proximal senses, the following section looks at how treatment can be designed for children who have sensory integration problems in each of these specific areas. The treatment ideas which follow are those that have been used in clinical practice and have been shown to have positive results with children. Even though they have been divided into sections covering proprioceptive, vestibular and tactile activities, all activities will influence the three sensory systems, as they do not function in isolation.

When carrying out the following input, be sure to notice if the child appears to 'switch off'. This is known as 'sensory shut down' and occurs when the sensory system is overloaded, and is unable to integrate and organise effectively all of the incoming sensory information.

Proprioceptive input

Handling techniques used in neuro-development treatment, as described in chapter 5, will help to improve proprioceptive feedback by changing abnormal tone and facilitating more normal patterns of movement. Position and movement activities that encourage mobile weight-bearing are particularly good. The techniques of 'tapping' and 'compression' will also help to increase information to the joints.

The effect of better integration of proprioceptive sensation should give the child:

- A calming influence on the sensory system.
- More possibility of organising movements.
- Improved directional control of movements.
- A better repertoire of more varied movements.
- Better emotional security.
- More normal muscle tone.
- Improved body awareness.
- A more stable level of alertness and arousal.

Activity ideas to increase proprioceptive awareness

- Place the child on her front over a therapy ball or roll, so that she is supporting herself with her arms. Making sure she is in alignment, support her around the pelvis and lower back, and rock her gently back and forth to slightly increase the pressure through her arms.

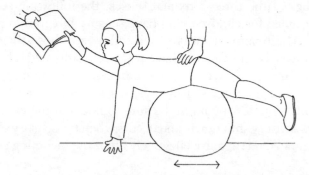

Figure 8.2

In this position, if there is a parent or other adult available, games can be played that involve reaching with one arm. Some examples are popping bubbles, collecting ingredients to make a play sandwich, batting a soft ball, picture card matching, and turning the pages of a storybook. As this can be an effortful activity, it is advisable to carefully grade the amount of time it is carried out and ensure that postural tone is not increasing in other parts of the body due to increased effort.

- Position the child face down in a hammock or on a platform swing (if available). Make sure he is in alignment. If he has difficulty relaxing at his hips, a soft roll can be placed under them to provide further support and help him feel more comfortable. He may also require a V-shaped cushion or long roll under his upper body.

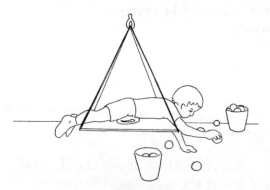

Figure 8.3

Encourage the child to use his arms to move himself in different directions, forward and backward, round and round. Play games such as collecting food for an aeroplane journey, going shopping, collecting the pieces of a puzzle or cards to make a picture story. These activities can be fun and will help to develop better movement planning and spatial awareness.

- Using a low swing or platform swing, sit the child with his feet in alignment on the ground. (It may be necessary to support the child at his knees to maintain alignment.) A similar action can be achieved over a roll or in a rocking chair. Encourage him to push forwards and backwards through his legs. If using a platform swing, incorporate turning by encouraging the child to side-step while he is holding onto the supporting ropes.

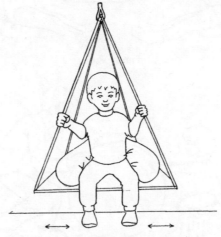

Figure 8.4

- Invite the child to lie on her front on a scooter board and use her arms to pull and move herself around an obstacle course. This not only helps improve proprioceptive awareness but also challenges a child's motor organisational and spatial perceptual planning skills. A supportive stretching belt may be necessary across her hips and bottom.

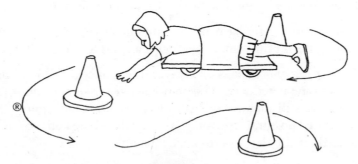

Figure 8.5

- Play a gentle game of pushing and pulling, or rowing a boat, sitting on a soft cushion with legs extended in front. This can also be carried out with children in wheelchairs, and in standing or high kneeling with a therapist supporting each child's hips.

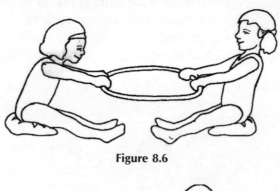

Figure 8.6

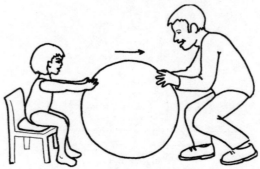

Figure 8.7

- In standing, sitting or high kneeling, play pushing games against a large therapy ball, hands on hands or up against the wall.

- Roll the child in a soft blanket and tap over her body. Swaddle young babies and children, if they tolerate it, and use heavy blankets for sleeping under.

- Using elasticated bands, cumba bands or kimono belts wrapped around the child's trunk, and tubi-grips on the arms, often helps a child to have better body awareness.

- Place sandbags or heavy beanbags on arms and legs once a child has gained a relaxed position and her tone is reduced. This is not active movement, but it gives the child time in a calm and still manner to better feel her limbs and joints. It also helps to maintain the reduced postural tone gained through handling and movement techniques, without the need for the therapist to be 'hands-on'.

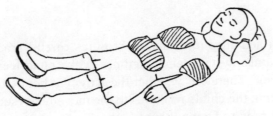

Figure 8.8

- Carefully position a young baby or child in a 'nested' position, giving consistent input to his head, arms and legs. A V-shaped pillow and rolls are very useful for this, but rolled up towels or blankets can also be used effectively.

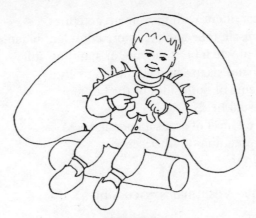

Figure 8.9

- Carry out activities such as banging a drum or tambourine, rolling out play dough, cooking, kneading plasticine and singing songs that involve finding and tapping body parts.

- Encourage scribbling, drawing or writing activities that use wax crayons, chalk on chalkboards, and weighted pencils. Weighted pencils can be made by sellotaping metal washers onto the pencil or by wrapping string curtain weights around them. Use crayons and chalks that need to be held in the palm of the hand, as these require larger movements of the whole arm, which further increases proprioceptive feeling.

- Introduce biting and chewing on firm, crunchy foods. Before suggesting this, *always* consult the speech and language therapist and, if one is not available, observe a child's eating and swallowing skills very carefully.

Vestibular input

Introducing movement activities into therapy requires careful grading and observation, since input to the vestibular system can sometimes evoke rapid feelings of nausea. It can also increase postural tone. Therefore, whether the activity is bouncing on a ball, rocking in a swing or sitting on a roll, the child's reactions to the movement (such as his postural tone or movement patterns) need to be monitored.

Combining proprioceptive with vestibular input helps the sensory system to integrate the feeling of motion more easily. It also gives the child a more consistent and regulated feeling about the position of his body in space, helping him to feel more secure.

Better integration of vestibular sensation should help the child to:

- Become calm and confident with movement activities.
- Gain more stable muscle tone and feel more confident when moving.
- Have a better sense of when he is moving or standing still.
- Be better orientated and secure in relation to gravity.
- Coordinate movements of both sides of the body.
- Maintain a stable visual field.
- Have a more balanced level of arousal and alertness.
- Have a clearer interpretation of other senses.

Activity ideas to improve vestibular processing

Vestibular hyposensitivity

Children with athetoid CP are those most frequently hyposensitive to vestibular input, and tend to enjoy high levels of movement. They often display poor central tone, affecting their ability to stabilise centrally, and making it harder to control graded moments of their arms and legs. Vestibular input helps increase central tone and also helps to reduce the range of fluctuating tone experienced with athetoid CP. Activities described in the section on proprioception can also be useful.

- Using a therapy ball, have the child sit with feet off the floor, giving deep pressure at the hips. Begin to bounce the ball, pressing firmly downwards. Give three to five strong bounces, then wait for the child to sit up and bring his arms down onto the ball. The aim is to increase active extension but to avoid extreme extension, as this throws the child backwards.

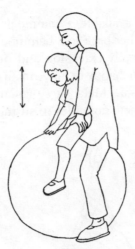

Figure 8.10

- The action of bouncing helps to increase a child's level of arousal and can help to reduce the fluctuations of postural tone. After using the ball it can be helpful to sit on a firm surface, for instance on a bench, or in supportive standing. The child may now be able both to focus his attention more on an activity and gain better control of his movements.
- An air-filled cushion can give a low-level, ongoing vestibular input to a child sitting in an ordinary chair. This can help him maintain better postural control and aid his arousal level.

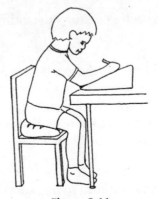

Figure 8.11

- Use a swing at the park or, if available, a hammock or platform swing. The child may choose to lie on her front or her back in a hammock or platform swing. Lying on her front will encourage upper body extension and help with hip extension. If a child likes to swing she may be quite happy to move in all directions and enjoy being pushed fairly high, so long as this is safe. Make sure regular breaks are given. After swinging, work on slow, graded movement activities in sitting or standing.

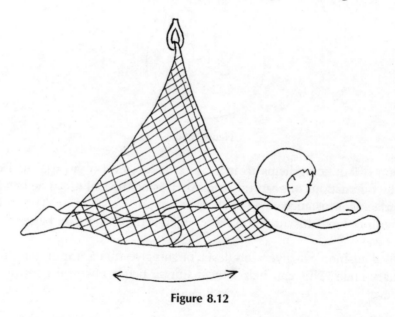

Figure 8.12

- Work regularly in positions such as sitting or standing, which are up against gravity.

Vestibular hypersensitivity

Children with increased postural tone, or those who have strong intermittent or dystonic spasms, often appear to be more sensitive to movement activities. Using movement in a graded and rhythmical way, combined with proprioceptive input, can help reduce their sensitivity to movement. It also improves their overall arousal level and helps them to relax their body, 'letting go' of positions and postures they may have fixed themselves into for the feeling of security.

- Place the child on her back on a platform swing, supported comfortably with cushions around her shoulders and under her knees. With your hands on her upper trunk and pelvis, gently move the swing forwards and backwards in a linear plane. Singing rhythmically or humming in time to the motion can help the child to be calm and get used to the movement.

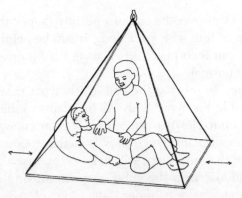

Figure 8.13

When the child's postural tone has come down, begin to move the child's limbs into better alignment, reducing positions of flexion and adduction. Use careful facilitation and handling. It may be difficult to gain symmetry and alignment for a child who is very dystonic, in which case slowly grade the change of her body position. Pay particular attention to the position of her head, as it is often turned strongly to one side. It may take longer, or a number of sessions, before you are able to place the head into a midline position.

• Place the child on her front over a large ball, perhaps with a soft roll under her upper trunk for comfort. With your hands on the upper and lower part of her body gently press down and release to give movement through the ball and a gentle sensation of bouncing for the child. If the child is comfortable with this, you can then alter the movement and move the ball in a linear, forward-and-backward direction. This will give the child a gentle rocking sensation. This activity can help reduce tone around the hips and within the leg muscles, so that they are easier to move, e.g., for positioning her in a standing frame.

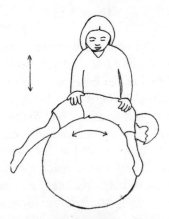

Figure 8.14

- Sit the child with his legs over the end of a peanut-shaped therapy ball, or roll, and sit behind him to support him with your body. It can be helpful to call the ball a bus, a bike or a boat. You can then make up an imaginary journey, in which movement is necessary and quite normal!

    Begin your journey by moving the ball gently from side to side, making sure the child feels supported in his upper body. As he adapts to the movement, his tone may reduce enough for you to slowly open out his legs far enough to place them on either side of the ball. This will enable you to slowly facilitate extension and alignment of his trunk. The action of the movement will help to increase the activity of the extensor muscles further, and also help the child adapt to moving out of his central base of support. As he becomes more confident, the range of side-to-side movement can be increased. Introduce some bouncing and very gradually reduce the degree of hands-on support. This may require a number of therapy sessions, depending on the child.

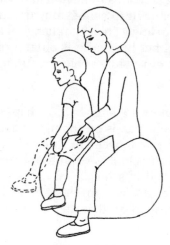

Figure 8.15

- To further upgrade the activity you can introduce some trunk rotation and reaching. Use equipment that helps the child to feel safe and comfortably positioned. A child who is fearful of moving out of her base of support or moving backwards may also have very poor trunk rotation. To help her develop active rotation, put her in a seat with sides for added security and with her feet firmly placed on the floor. A table that half-encircles the child will also make her feel safe. In this position, the child can begin to turn to the sides to play, as well as face forward. Put toys at the side of the table and behind her and encourage her to reach for them. Giving the child the security of the table to put her hands on helps reduces her anxiety, and from her own activity through play, moving and turning can become more integrated and automatic.

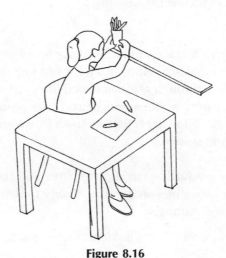

Figure 8.16

Tactile input

A child who has problems tolerating tactile stimulus needs a gradual introduction to different tactile sensations. The child should feel that she is playing and exploring while she experiences, over time, a variety of textures, objects and toys. This is the best way for her sensory system to integrate various sensations, to learn about size, shape and form, and to discriminate between textures.

However, it is also important to notice if the child becomes quickly overloaded by tactile sensory input, appearing to 'switch off'. This is known as 'sensory shut-down' and occurs when the sensory system is unable to integrate and organise effectively all of the incoming sensory information.

Better integration of tactile sensations can help the child to:

- Become more alert and calm for activities.
- Tolerate sensation better, for example of clothing and textured objects.
- Maintain arousal and concentration.
- Decrease or increase muscle tone.
- Develop early emotional well-being and feelings of security.
- Develop better oral control (for example, sucking and chewing).
- Achieve daily activities such as dressing, eating and washing.
- Have better body awareness.
- Develop the correct grasp and manipulation of objects.
- Interpret and remember tactile information, such as in holding a pencil.

Activity ideas to improve tactile processing

Touch hypersensitivity

Grade the child's contact with textures. Initially it may be enough to play next to the child with, for example, only toys that are soft or furry. Do not impose textures on the child, invite him to touch and explore through games and activities. Try to use toys and objects that vary in texture, combining firm wooden and plastic toys with soft and/or furry objects. When carrying out any of the following activities, use a firm touch, giving deep pressure, as this will help calm the tactile system.

- Introduce messy play gradually, starting with firm objects. For example, use rolling pins and cutters with plasticine, progressing slowly to flattening the plasticine on the tabletop with hard hand patting.

- Allow the child to find firm objects hidden in rice or sand.

- Give her 'feely boxes' with mainly firm toys and objects inside them, and only one or two soft or furry objects to incidentally touch.

- Use brushes or sponges with handles for painting. Progress slowly to finger-painting without imposing paint on the child's hand. Always have a cloth close by to wipe her hands. Use deep proprioceptive input when cleaning them.

- Encourage pretend activities, such as washing, dressing and grooming a doll, making cups of tea or playing with pretend food of various textures.

- Swaddle the child by rolling him in a soft blanket, and gently tap him to give firm proprioceptive and consistent tactile input.

- Remove labels from clothing and use soft fabrics, particularly for undergarments.

- With young babies, placing a soft muslin cloth over their limbs when handling them can help to reduce oversensitivity to touch.

- Babies and young children who are hypersensitive benefit from being wrapped and carried on their mother's back. This practice, common in African and South American countries, helps give the child who is hypersensitive input to all three systems: tactile, proprioceptive *and* vestibular. The combination is a very integrating experience for the baby.

Touch hyposensitivity

- Combine deep proprioceptive input—such as tapping and deep stroking—with handling the child.

- During bath and wash time use a body mitt, and give extra-deep rubbing with the towel to dry.

- Encourage playing and manipulating firm, hard objects, as this will give more consistent tactile information than soft-textured toys. Incorporate a variety of tactile activities during play. For instance:

  - Wet and dry sand play.
  - Painting with hands, sponges and clothes.
  - Water play with variously textured objects and toys.
  - Plasticine; hide objects in the plasticine to find.
  - Feeling objects with eyes closed, describing and naming them if possible.
  - Exploring a tin full of objects with the same shape but different texture, such as small balls of different types.
  - Playing with toys that vibrate.

- Give the child time to play in minimal clothing.

- Specific oral-facial therapy can be very beneficial; this can be discussed with the speech and language therapist. Also refer to the section on 'Managing problems of sensation' in chapter 9.

- Adapt tools; use pencils with textured grippers; give a selection of variously sized and shaped pencils and crayons. Give cutlery with moulded *and* shaped handles.

Children cared for in an institution

Children with CP who do not have parents or regular carers to look after them need a particularly sensitive and consistent approach. The way they are handled is important. Careful positioning is essential, not only to maintain postural alignment and prevent contractures and deformity, but also to help the children feel safe and secure. Giving regular rhythmical motion can also help them develop regulatory states, such as establishing a sleep–wake cycle, having times for feeling hungry, and the ability to control emotional responses. These are necessary for sleeping and self-calming. The absence of these regulatory states makes it difficult for children who are cared for within an institution to develop their ability to process tactile, proprioceptive and vestibular information, because they lack the regular experiences received through day-to-day parental love, touch and attention. Giving them the opportunity for more appropriate sensory experiences allows their nervous systems to better integrate those sensations they may have difficulty with.

CASE STUDIES

Rami

Observations

Rami is a delightful 4-year-old boy who is very animated, communicative and likes to be engaged in play. He was born very pre-term at 24 weeks and has severe dystonic athetoid CP. His dystonic spasms are so frequent and strong that he is unable to hold any posture for long, and his head is constantly turned to the right no matter what position he is in.

Rami has difficulty sleeping because his body pushes into an overextended posture, and he becomes distressed when he finds himself 'stuck' in this position. It is also extremely difficult for Rami's parents to position him comfortably, to play with him, and for Rami to concentrate and hold his attention on books, games and other activities. He cannot relax his own body and 'let go' of fixed end-of-range positions, which are not functional or comfortable for him.

Conclusions

The therapist concluded that, along with other difficulties, Rami could be hyposensitive to proprioceptive information. The frequent spasms and movement make it very difficult for Rami to gain a consistent feeling of his body and its position. His pushing and finding strong end-of-range postures could be due to his need to gain this feedback.

Treatment

The aim of Rami's treatment is to teach him to relax himself, using the sensation of deep pressure to help him experience a more consistent body awareness. This should help him to bring his head into a midline position without hands-on facilitation. The therapist used two different approaches:

- Lying Rami on his back on a platform swing, with support from a V-shaped pillow and a soft roll under his knees (see Figure 8.14). As the therapist moved the swing forward and backwards rhythmically with one hand on Rami's chest, he was able to gradually relax from his fixed position, although his body remained twisted. The therapist was then able to gradually place him in an aligned position with his head in midline. Although he continued to push his body into an extended position, he was more able to relax himself without the therapist facilitating.

- Placing weighted bags on his chest, shoulders and thighs (see Figure 8.8) to give him very clear pro-prioceptive feedback. This had an immediate effect. With no hands-on facilitation, Rami relaxed his body and turned his head to a midline position by himself. (Usually, bringing Rami's head to midline would have created a strong reaction in his whole body, causing twisting and extending.) He was able to remain comfortably in an aligned posture while a story was read to him, smiling and relaxed, keeping his attention throughout.

The weighted bags give Rami a strong proprioceptive sensation and this seems to be enough to stop him from needing to seek out and fix in end-of-range positions. Rami's response to having the weighted bags placed on him has been consistent. Although it is not an active posture, we have found a way for Rami to remain still and calm, using his eyes to explore pictures while listening to and enjoying a story. Here, Rami can also communicate using his eyes and facial expressions without his whole body extending. It has been thrilling for Rami's parents to read him a story without needing to hold or frequently reposition him.

Sena

Observations
Sena is an 8-year-old boy who has choreo-athetosis with wide-ranging movement. He has very good motor organisational skills and can automatically plan the direction and combinations of his movements. He also has a good understanding of spatial direction, knowing the movements, directions and line combination necessary for him to form his letters and numbers. Sena attends a mainstream school and both his parents and teachers recognise that he has a high level of ability. Despite being a very active boy, however, his underlying low postural tone and the fluctuation of his muscle tone make it very difficult for him to hold himself in any position for long without support. As a result he finds it hard to hold his attention, or to grade and control his movements. This poor attention and constant need to change position affects his learning. For instance, Sena wanted to learn to drive a powered wheelchair and develop better control of the joystick on his school computer, but was struggling to practise these activities due to his movement activity, level of excitement and limited concentration.

Conclusions
The therapist observed Sena's constant need to move, over and above the movement caused by his fluctuating muscle tone. She sensed that he could be hyposensitive to vestibular information, requiring extra amounts of movement in order to satisfy the needs of his sensory system. This is common for children with this type of CP.

Treatment
The therapist felt that if his need for movement was better satisfied, Sena might find it easier to hold his concentration and develop more graded and organised movement control. She decided to use a hammock to give Sena the opportunity to experience free and varied

movements. She chose a hammock held by a single hook, as it gives better range and direction than a hammock fixed at both ends.

- Lying on his front, Sena was encouraged to move himself around by pushing with his arms. This kind of movement increases the proprioceptive information in the arms, which helps to improve upper-body stability and body awareness. Once he was used to moving himself around in the hammock, Sena was invited to go 'flying'. The therapist pulled him by his outstretched arms, then released, to let him swing freely with lifted arms. Sena had to use active upper-body extension to hold up his arms and head, while enjoying the experience of motion. This exercise alone helps develop the active trunk activity and extension which is very necessary for Sena. Once he has tired of this position he can roll over onto his back and continue to swing, this time with a circular motion. He can experience this movement repeatedly without getting dizzy, another indication of his hypo-responsiveness to vestibular activity.

- After swinging in the hammock, Sena was happier, calmer and had fewer involuntary movements. This means he is better able to concentrate, and happier to try the activities he usually finds challenging. Immediately after swinging, Sena was positioned on his front, supporting himself with one arm and with a sheet of paper in front of him on an upright board. He was able to work in a more focused and controlled way on his handwriting. Following the activity in the hammock, Sena was also able to sit for a short time by himself in a regular chair, holding himself upright in a more controlled and stable position than was possible prior to using the hammock.

Sena now shows better directional control with his hands, and his focus on letter formation is improving.

Eva

Observations

Eva is a 4-year-old girl with a diagnosis of spastic diplegia. She also has markedly increased tone in her left arm, though no abnormal tone in her right. Eva is a very chatty and happy little girl, who is determined to be independent in her daily activities. She has received physiotherapy and occupational therapy since she was 1 year old, and has always been very tolerant of the exercises and play activities. Eva was very keen to walk, but at this stage she was unable to support herself well enough with a walking aid. Eva's physiotherapist suggested instead that she try riding a little tricycle. At about the same time, her mother started to encourage Eva to use the toilet.

However, when the therapist tried to move her both on a tricycle and on a therapy ball, with very small, gentle motions, Eva became extremely distressed. Her mother also noticed that Eva became rigid, fearful and upset when she was put on the toilet, even though she wanted to use it like her sister.

Conclusions

Such a rapid reaction to movement when well supported indicated that Eva might be experiencing a degree of gravitational insecurity, the fear of movement due to vestibular hypersensitivity. The therapist was aware of her postural insecurity, but Eva's reactions were clearly out of proportion to the degree of movement and level of support she was given. Her reaction to moving slightly backwards on a therapy ball was a clear indication that she was experiencing gravitational insecurity. This affects many aspects of a child's daily function—along with reduced postural control and poor saving reactions, any movement or positions without stability can make her very fearful.

Treatment

The aim of Eva's treatment was to overcome her fears by using movement in a very gradual, gentle way. Eva was placed on a peanut-shaped therapy ball, with the therapist sitting behind her to support her around the trunk, with her hands on Eva's knees. The therapist played a game of being on a rowboat, slowly rocking the ball from side to side. Gradually, she added a small amount of gentle bouncing while singing a song with Eva. Eva gradually began to relax, her trunk activity improved, and it became possible for her to relax her legs enough to place them on either side of the ball. During the first session Eva became slightly more confident, and the therapist was able to increase the degree of motion slightly, while maintaining the same degree of postural support. Eva had treatment on a weekly basis and gradually the level of movement increased, with bouncing and rocking motions. The therapist pretended that the ball was a bicycle on which Eva was cycling down the hill, or a boat on the calm sea which became a little rocky at times, or a horse trotting gently along, speeding up to a canter. Since the movement activities were fun, imaginary and gentle, Eva entered into the feeling of playfulness which helped her to be happy and relaxed. Eva's confidence changed during the sessions, so that she enjoyed sitting on the therapy ball. Her mother also noticed a great difference when she put Eva on the toilet, and she was happy to try riding the tricycle again. Working with gentle and graded movement in a playful way helped improve Eva's very sensitive vestibular processing, reducing her fear and helping her to feel more confident.

Libbie

Observations

Libbie is a 6-month-old baby who experienced a severe physical trauma at 17 days old. As a result she is brain damaged, and has CP affecting her whole body. Libbie began receiving therapy at 3 months. From the outset she clearly was very sensitive to any touch or tactile experience. This affected her positioning, handling, dressing and feeding. Her sensitivity seemed particularly acute in the palms of her hands, around her lips and within her mouth. She had a tendency to hold her hands fisted, but this was not due to increased postural tone, as she can spontaneously open her hands with a normal and effortless movement pattern.

When fed with a bottle, Libbie screams for up to five minutes. Once she has accommodated to the sensation of the milk, she settles down, and is able to suckle and swallow very well. This pattern occurs every time she is fed. Libbie's carer is very careful with her positioning during feeding, and uses a consistent, graded and gentle approach to ensure Libbie feels secure and is able to feed well. Libbie's carer began to introduce her to semi-solid food at the recommendation of the speech and language therapist. As with the milk, when the food touched Libbie's lips she screamed and was unable to accommodate to the sensation of the texture within her mouth.

Conclusions

Libbie's speech and language therapist felt that her problem was due to a tactile sensory problem and asked the occupational therapist's opinion. In a joint session, they carefully observed Libbie's response to eating and drinking. They noticed that Libbie's reaction to careful tactile information on her hands was identical to the reaction when food touched the skin around and within her mouth. They concluded that Libbie was experiencing a tactile modulation difficulty, with hypersensitivity of her tactile system.

Treatment

The aim of Libbie's treatment was to improve her processing of tactile information.

The therapists recommended that Libbie's carer give gentle but deep pressure when touching Libbie's hands. She should open Libbie's hands and place them on each other, on Libbie's own face and around her mouth. We also suggested that with open hands Libbie is encouraged to feel and touch her own clothing and blanket and play with a variety of textured toys. Libbie's carer should always incorporate firm touch with those that had a soft texture.

To improve Libbie's oral sensitivity, the sensitivity of her hands needed to be worked on at the same time, as the sensory experience of the hands and mouth are closely linked. To help her tolerate solid foods, the therapists recommended giving her a gentle but quite firm finger massage around the outside of her mouth, with the pressure directed downward above her top lip and upward at the bottom lip. Her carer began feeding her by placing a small amount of food on the back of Libbie's hand, gradually bringing it up to her mouth for her to begin to touch, feel and suck. We suggested this be carried out daily.

After two weeks of Libbie's carer carrying out these ideas, Libbie is able to take her milk from the bottle without screaming. She is happy to have her hands massaged and touched, and does not react strongly. Libbie is starting to bat and play with firm toys, opening her fingers quite spontaneously. She is not yet able to tolerate the more solid foods, either on her lips or inside her mouth; however, her carer is confident that this will improve over time, and is continuing with the recommendations that were made initially.

EXAMPLES OF USEFUL EQUIPMENT

- *Therapy ball*, in round or peanut shape. The size to use will depend on the age and size of the child. Where a therapy ball is not available, a large inner tube may work instead.
- A *roll*. This can be made out of large tin cans, approximately 15 cm wide and 25 cm high, joined together and then covered with layers of foam or soft padding.
- A *therapeutic platform swing*. This can be made from a strong piece of flat, hard wood. The dimensions can be altered to accommodate space. A useful dimension is 60 × 115 cm, with cushioned edges and a rug or carpet on the base. Strong ropes should be attached to each corner of the platform. The ropes can be attached centrally to a strong metal ring, which can then be hung on a robust metal hook fixed securely into a ceiling joist.
- A *hammock*, fixed at two points or fixed at one (see Figure 8.13).

Note: All suspended equipment *must* be checked for safety.

- *Wobble board*. This is a wooden board, approximately 50 × 80 cm in size, with half-circle castors at either end to give stability but enable the platform base to move gently from side to side.
- *Scooter board*. This can be made from a flat piece of hard wood approximately 40 × 80 cm in size (this can be varied), covered in a soft foam or fabric, with a castor at each corner.
- *Vibration toys*, such as a vibrating snake or cushion.
- *Soft V-shaped pillow*, *medium-sized rolls* and *long sausage rolls*.
- *Elasticated* or *lycra band* or a *kimono band*.
- *Soft muslin* cloth.
- *Firm toys*, including drums, rattles, cause-and-effect pop-up toys, plastic buckets and wooden blocks.
- *Body mitt*.
- *Sandbags* or *weighted bean bags* of various sizes, 20 × 20 cm, 10 × 10 cm and 10 × 5 cm, according to the size of the child.

REFERENCES

Anderson, J. 1996. 'Sensory Intervention with the Preterm Infant in the Neonatal Intensive Care Unit'. *The American Journal of Occupational Therapy*, 40(1), January.

Ayres, A.J. 1979. *Sensory Integration and the Child*. Los Anngeles: Western Psychological Services.

Battaile, B., G. DeGangi, T. Long and A. Wiener. 1996. 'Sensory Processing of Infants Born Prematurely or with Regulatory Disorders'. *Physical & Occupational Therapy in Pediatrics*, 16(4).

Blanche, E.I. 2000. Sensory Integration Therapy and Children with CP: Course Notes.

Blanche, E.I., T.M. Botticelli and M.K. Hallway. 1995. *Combining Neuro-developmental Treatment and Sensory Integration Principles: An Approach to Pediatric Therapy*. Tucson, AZ: Therapy Skill Builders.

Bobath course notes 1998: Bobath Centre London.

DeGangi, G.A. 2000. Advanced Course in Assessing Young Children with Multisensory, Interactional and Attentional Problems: Course Notes.

————. 1994. *Documenting Sensorimotor Progress: A Pediatric Therapist's Guide*. Tucson, AZ: Therapy Skill Builders.

Fisher, A.G., E.A. Murry and A.C. Bundy. 1991. *Sensory Integration: Theory and Practice*. Philadelphia: F.A. Davis.

Lesny, I., A. Stehlik, J. Tomasek, A. Tomankova and I. Havlicek. 1993. 'Sensory Disorders in Cerebral Palsy: Two Point Discrimination'. *Developmental Medicine and Child Neurology*, 35(5): 402–405.

Moore, J. 1984. 'The Neuroanatomy and Pathology of CP'. *Neurodevelopmental Treatment Association Newsletter*, May.

Oetter, P., E.W. Richter and S.M. Frick. 2001. *M.O.R.E. Integrating the Mouth with Sensory and Postural Functions*, 2nd edition. Hugo, MN: PDP Press.

Roley, S.S., E.I. Blanche and R.C. Schaaf, eds. 2001. *Understanding the Nature of Sensory Integration with Diverse Populations*. San Antonio, TX: Therapy Skill Builders.

Stock Kranowitz, C. 1998. *The Out-of-Sync Child: Recognizing and Coping with Sensory Integration Dysfunction*. New York: Perigee Book.

ANNIE BROZAITIS has 15 years' experience as a paediatric occupational therapist. She worked for two years developing a paediatric OT service in Bolivia, South America, and three years at the Bobath Centre in Cardiff, Wales. She is currently working in Community Paediatrics at Frenchay Hospital in Bristol, England. Annie's specialist skill is in working with babies and young children who have cerebral palsy. Her particular interest is in combining the theory and approaches of the Bobath concept with those of sensory integration therapy.

Chapter 9

Assessment and management of eating and drinking difficulties

MARIAN BROWNE

INTRODUCTION

MANY children with cerebral palsy have eating and drinking difficulties These range from relatively minor difficulties in coordination of oral movements causing eating to be slow and with excessive spillage, to severe incoordination of the swallowing mechanism, causing ill health and even life-threatening conditions. Mealtimes may take up to 15 times longer than for other children (Gisel and Patrick 1988), and despite this the children often do not receive adequate nourishment. A community-based study by Reilly et al. (1996) revealed oral-motor problems in more than 90 per cent of a sample of 49 children with cerebral palsy, of whom over a third were at risk of chronic undernourishment.

For most of us, eating and drinking is a pleasure, and an important opportunity to meet socially with friends and family. Feeding times form a vital part of the bonding process which occurs between the mother and the young infant. As the child grows, mealtimes provide opportunities to learn communication and social skills. The child with cerebral palsy who has difficulty eating may have very negative experiences of eating and drinking. Carers are often anxious about ensuring adequate food and water intake for their child, and this anxiety frequently interferes with healthy communication and feeding practices. Experiences of coughing and choking may be frequent and very frightening for many children with eating difficulties, and for their carers. It is common for children to show a strong aversion to food and drink. In addition, as many as 70 per cent of children with severe neurological impairment experience some degree of gastro-oesophageal reflux, which itself may cause chronic and severe pain (Reyas et al. 1993) and contribute to food refusal and respiratory tract infections.

Eating and drinking problems are often found to be the major cause of concern for parents of children with cerebral palsy. If managed poorly, they may worsen over time and cause ill health (Cass et al. 2005). However, appropriate handling of children at mealtimes and careful management of food and feeding techniques can minimise these harmful symptoms and sometimes prevent them from occurring (Evans Morris and Dunn Klein 2000; Larnert and Ekberg 1995; Gisel et al. 1996).

THE DEVELOPMENT OF EATING AND DRINKING

In order to recognise and understand difficulties in eating and drinking, it is important to have a sound understanding of the normal processes involved, and the way in which eating and drinking skills develop in the young infant and child. Parents will recognise that the well-being of young babies is dependent on the quality of their feeding: how readily they take milk, how much they take at a time, whether they have indigestion, 'colic' or reflux and whether they can establish a regular pattern of feeding and sleeping. Difficulties at this stage may be the first indication of an abnormality in the developmental process.

There are a number of significant differences between the oral–pharyngeal anatomy of newborns and that of adults (Evans Morris and Dunn Klein 2000). These differences support the infants' ability to swallow safely until about 3 or 4 months of age and include the following:

1. The newborn's intraoral space is small.
2. The lower jaw is small and slightly retracted.
3. Sucking pads are present in the newborn.
4. The tongue takes up relatively more space in the mouth of the newborn.
5. The tongue moves in a more restricted way.
6. Newborns prefer to breathe through the nose.
7. The epiglottis and soft palate are in close approximation in the newborn as a protective mechanism.
8. The larynx is higher in the neck of the newborn reducing the need for laryngeal closure to protect the airway during swallowing.
9. The hyoid is made of cartilage (not bone) in the infant.
10. The Eustachian tube lies in a more horizontal position in the infant.

These differences diminish after 4 months, making possible the development of a more mature eating and drinking pattern. However, where neurological maturation is impaired, the reduction of anatomical protection at this stage may leave the child vulnerable to eating difficulties and aspiration.

The normal eating and drinking process is made possible by the presence of a number of protective and adaptive responses which include coughing, gagging, sucking, swallowing and chewing.

Adaptive responses

Babies are known to swallow from the twelfth week of gestation or earlier (Humphrey 1970). The healthy baby is usually able to locate a nipple or teat by his *rooting reflex*. This enables the baby to turn his mouth to the source of touch on his face, and to latch on to it to begin sucking. Although there is great variation in the way in which babies suck and swallow, healthy babies are able to suck in a rhythmical pattern, and to coordinate this with regular breathing. Although some coughing may occur, it is very occasional. The coordination of sucking, breathing and swallowing is smooth, and the baby automatically stops breathing momentarily during a swallow. Immediately after a swallow, the infant breathes out, clearing any slight residue from the airway. The speed and strength of sucking will be determined by the baby's degree of hunger, level of arousal, milk supply and so on.

The *suck–swallow response* is usually elicited by rooting. The infant moves his tongue vigorously in a forward-and-backward pattern and swallows regularly after each suck. From about 3 months this pattern is gradually modified to a more mature suck which involves elevation of the tongue tip. The baby begins to be able to swallow without a prior suck.

Protective responses

There are two protective responses, the cough and the gag, which are present at birth. The *gag reflex* prevents the baby from taking anything too large or otherwise dangerous into the digestive system and causes the tongue and pharyngeal muscles to eject the food forwards into the mouth (a kind of reverse peristalsis). The *cough reflex* is triggered by something actually entering the airway or blocking the entrance to it. It causes a sharp breath outwards to expel the foreign material or buildup of secretions. The cough reflex is the body's most important protection for the airway during eating and drinking.

Weaning

In the Western world, from 4 to 5 months, babies are introduced to semi-solid or puréed food on a spoon. The baby is placed in a sitting position where the head is fully supported and stable. Initially, food is sucked from the spoon with a forward-and-backward tongue movement, in the process of which quite a lot of food may be pushed out of the mouth. The feeder helps the baby remove the food from the spoon by tipping the spoon up. Gradually, the baby's tongue starts to move in a more upward-and-downward direction in the mouth, and the lips become more effective in removing food from the spoon.

From 3 months, babies begin to enjoy putting their own hands in their mouths. Soon they are able to hold toys and clothes to their mouths too, and by approximately 5 months, many babies also enjoy sucking their own toes. For the majority of waking hours, the infant explores the environment through this 'mouthing' process which plays an important part in the development of self-awareness and body image. It is recognised to be an important part of the development of oral skills, and through this process children develop control of their tongue, lips and jaw, and learn to recognise a variety of different sensations.

By 6 months, the infant is beginning to sit and is developing good head control. This provides the essential *stability* that makes possible the development of chewing and babbling. When the head is stable, the infant's tongue can begin to move separately from the jaw and more complex patterns of mouth movements are possible.

The beginnings of *chewing* can be seen at about 5 months. To begin with, pressure on the infant's gums elicits a regular up-and-down biting or 'munching' pattern on a hard toy or fingers. If something is placed to the sides of the mouth, the tongue will move to touch it by a kind of 'rooting'. Once a piece of food is softened by munching, it moves onto the centre of the tongue and can be sucked. At this stage it is not safe to give a baby hard foods to chew, since small pieces of solid food in the mouth may cause choking.

The baby's ability to move the tongue sideways increases, and from 7 to 9 months, a rotatory movement of the jaw can be seen when food is held in the mouth. At first, the food is 'held' between the teeth and hands are used to break the food into manageable pieces. By 12 months the baby can use the tongue to move food from the centre to the sides of the mouth for chewing. By 2 years, a hard bite can be sustained with the jaw. The head may still be tilted and hands used to break off something very hard, such as a piece of carrot.

As the young baby develops, the use of the lips to actively remove food from a spoon becomes more apparent. By 18 months, chewing with the lips closed (to keep all the food in the mouth) is possible, although some spillage and dribbling is common up to about 2 years. The occurrence of mouth closure during chewing tends to be determined by the cultural environment. During swallowing, the lips are closed from early infancy.

The introduction of babies to *drinking* from a cup varies enormously, although for many in Western Europe, it begins at the same time as the introduction of semi-solid food. Cups with a spout are usually used at first so that the baby can use the forward-backward sucking pattern effectively to take fluid from the cup. The tongue may protrude beneath the cup to provide some stability, and then the child may learn to bite on the edge of the cup to keep it stable. As the child's control of lip and jaw movements develops, the flow of fluid from an open cup is controlled by lips. By 2 years, a more mature drinking pattern is apparent; the jaw is held still without biting the cup and the tongue moves in a more up-and-down sucking pattern.

NORMAL EATING AND DRINKING PATTERNS

In order to recognise and effectively treat eating and drinking problems, we need to understand the way in which we normally take food into our mouths, chew and swallow it. It is helpful to consider this process in three stages: the pre-oral stage, the oral stage and the swallow.

The pre-oral stage

Before we take food into our mouths we normally have our mouths lightly closed, with jaw and lips together, but with no contact between the teeth. The tongue rests in the lower jaw, possibly lightly touching the teeth. Saliva production is minimal and we swallow the saliva we produce regularly, but without thinking about it. The breathing pattern is relatively slow, deep and rhythmical.

As the food approaches the mouth, there would usually be a slight increase in the amount of saliva produced. The lips purse or move forward slightly, and the lower jaw opens just enough to allow the food to be placed in the mouth. This graded movement of the lips and jaw is regulated finely and timed perfectly to 'greet' the approaching food, as we monitor visually the food intake. The lips seal around the food to control intake, and hold it in as the utensil is removed, or as we bite food off. The intake of food into the mouth is usually preceded by inspiration and then followed by expiration, thereby minimising the possibility of breathing food down into the airway.

The oral stage

Once the food is in our mouths, we keep our heads in a stable position. The chin is tucked in and the back of the neck is always elongated to give the airway the maximum protection against food going down the wrong way. Whatever position the body assumes, standing, sitting or reclining, elongation of the back of the neck is maintained because it is essential for safety in swallowing.

Food in the mouth is controlled by the tongue, cheeks and lips working together. The inside of the mouth has fine sensory awareness, which enables the tongue to locate food, move it to the sides and keep it between the teeth for chewing. Chewing usually comprises a mixture of up-and-down, side-to-side and rotatory jaw movements. If the texture of food is mixed, we swallow the runny components, and then chew the remaining more solid material. These selective movements of the tongue, lips and jaw all depend on the jaw being stable, and able to act as a support for the finely graded movements that are needed for chewing.

If the texture and quantity of food in the mouth require it, we may close our lips during chewing to prevent food or fluid from falling out. This use of our lips depends on sensory feedback from within and around the mouth. Breathing patterns are carefully regulated during eating so that we will usually exhale after taking food into the mouth as a safety measure against any particles being inhaled into the airway.

The swallow

When food is ready to be swallowed, we close our lips, and suck the food onto the centre of the tongue. Once food is held on the tongue, with lips still closed, we push it to the back of the mouth by lifting up the tongue tip, and then gradually the body of the tongue. When food reaches the back of the tongue, the pressure of the food on the sides of the pharynx triggers off the swallow reflex which ensures that the airway is protected as food passes over the entrance to the larynx, and that breathing momentarily stops.

ASSESSMENT OF EATING AND DRINKING PATTERNS IN THE CHILD WITH CEREBRAL PALSY

The presence of abnormal tone and altered oral sensory awareness in the child with cerebral palsy gives rise to typical abnormal eating and drinking patterns. These patterns can be understood by analysing the nature and distribution of postural tone. Appropriate management through handling, variation of the nature of food and fluid given, and therapeutic feeding techniques can then be implemented in accordance with this analysis.

It is helpful to look at typical problems which can be recognised in the three stages described above.

1. Pre-oral stage

Children who have eating and drinking difficulties may often feel anxious about mealtimes. Eating may be associated with excessive bouts of coughing or choking, which are frightening. In many cases where children suffer from gastro-oesophageal reflux (food coming up from the stomach), eating may be painful. Many children with severe eating difficulties may never be able to eat enough to satisfy their hunger.

The approach of food to the mouth, or the mere presentation of it before the child, may cause a significant increase in the occurrence of abnormal patterns of movement. The presentation of food arouses all the senses: vision, hearing, smell and touch, in addition to the emotions. This high level of stimulation may cause an increase in postural tone, involuntary movements, or the occurrence of spasms, and this in turn will impede the functional process of eating or drinking.

The following should all be assessed.

Position

Evaluation of the child's position is perhaps the most important part of the clinician's assessment of the eating and drinking process. The position of the child is the central factor which influences all other aspects of eating and drinking.

Is the child supported in a stable sitting or standing position? Is the trunk sufficiently stable to support the head? Is the spine extended and well aligned (not curving to one side)? Can the child maintain an elongated back of the neck during the eating and drinking process, or can this position be facilitated by handling and/or provision of supportive equipment?

It is important that the child and carer are comfortable at mealtimes and that the position assumed should not require constant effort to sustain. It is also important for the child to be able to monitor the approach of food visually, and to be able to make eye contact with the person assisting during the meal. Vision plays an important role in the accurate control of the timing and grading of jaw, lip and tongue movements in taking food or fluid into the mouth.

Jaw

Does the jaw provide a stable basis for movements of the tongue, cheeks and lips? How does it move and why does it move in this way?

Where increased tone is apparent, the jaw may be retracted (pulled back), associated with extension of the neck. If there is severe spasticity, the jaw may hardly open or move at all. It may open too far (compare to the opening of our mouths which is exactly graded to the size of food that is to be eaten). Where tone is low or fluctuating, the jaw may open and close excessively and thrust forwards. In some cases it may be pulled to one side or the other in association with increases in tone, or in cases of excessive involuntary movements. A bite reflex, which is an involuntary sustained biting action on something that touches the child's front teeth, may be extremely distressing and painful for the child. This may occur in children whose mouths are very sensitive and whose tone increases sharply as a result of tactile stimulation.

Lips

Is the child able to use the lips to remove food from a spoon, control fluid pouring from a cup or keep food in the mouth? If the lips are passive (not moving enough), then it is important to know the reason for this. Is the tone in the lips high or low? It is usually necessary to feel the lips to find this out. Can the child actually feel the food with the lips? In many cases the mouth opens too wide for the lips to respond to the presence of food; that is to say, the lips are unable to function adequately due to a lack of jaw stability which would normally give them a stable basis from which to work.

Tongue

Where does the tongue lie in the mouth when at rest? Can the tongue be still? Is it pulled upwards and back, or to one side in association with increased tone? Often, the tongue moves forwards and backwards in conjunction with the opening and closing of the jaw. This may sometimes be described as a 'tongue thrust' when the tongue protrudes beyond the lips. It may occur when there is no food in the mouth, for example in anticipation of food or drink, and will be more marked when the child uses effort. This pattern of tongue movement stems from a lack of stability of the jaw.

Can the tongue move food to the sides of the mouth in order for it to be chewed? In many cases the tongue moves only from front to back, and lacks lateral movements.

As a child prepares to eat or drink, there is normally an increase in saliva production. The child who has oral-motor control problems may have difficulty controlling this saliva in the mouth, and may start to dribble or cough. If the child coughs or aspirates saliva, anxiety may be constantly associated with eating and drinking. This in turn may cause the child's tone to increase or become more unstable, which will make swallowing even more difficult.

The most important area to assess when a child is eating and drinking is the coordination between *swallowing* and *breathing*. Many children with cerebral palsy habitually breathe through their mouths, rather than through their noses. The pattern of breathing may be irregular due to the occurrence of spasms or involuntary movements. When food or drink is presented to the child, they are therefore at much greater risk of *aspiration* (food going into the airway), which can cause chest infections or pneumonia. Eating and drinking is a finely tuned process of coordination which may easily be disturbed by changes in tone.

Symptoms of aspiration

When observing a child eating or drinking it is important to assess what happens when they swallow. Many indications of aspiration can be heard, such as noisy breathing (the sound of needing to clear the throat), coughing and prolonged apnoeas (when breathing stops). Other indications of aspiration may include blinking, blueness around the child's mouth, gagging or vomiting, and a look of fear or anxiety on the child's face. The child may make many attempts to initiate a swallow, and the swallow may only partially clear the oropharynx.

Aspiration is often a *silent* event and careful observation or investigation may be required to detect it. In some children there is a delay in the triggering of the swallow reflex, by which time some of food may already have fallen into the opening of the airway (a delayed swallow). Symptoms of aspiration may occur only when the child eats one particular texture. For example, many children are able to swallow soft, puréed foods safely, but when given water, which is more difficult to control, they may choke on it. The absence, when expected, of protective responses such as the cough can indicate that there is a high risk of aspiration occurring. All symptoms of aspiration are a serious cause for concern and indicate that therapy is needed for the child's safety and health (Cass et al. 2005; Morton et al. 1999). Intervention to minimise aspiration and thereby preserve the health of the child can be highly effective.

Oral sensory awareness

Sensation plays a very big role in determining a child's motor coordination in relation to eating and drinking. Normal motor responses require the brain to receive sensory information and to process or interpret an appropriate amount of such information. Difficulties in the reception, selection and perception of sensory information during eating and drinking can seriously affect the child's motor responses, and this in turn further affects the sensory processes (Evans Morris and Dunn Klein 2000).

Oral sensory awareness and perception is often disturbed in children who have abnormal postural tone, and this is an important area to evaluate. It is widely recognised that many children are hypersensitive to stimulation around and inside their mouths, but there are also many who are hyposensitive to oral stimulation. The two problems may superficially look similar. Both types of sensory disturbance may put the child at risk of aspiration when eating and drinking, and may worsen without intervention.

Hypersensitivity: The child has a stronger reaction to sensory stimulation than one would expect, or the reaction is more rapid. The sensory threshold is lowered.

Hyposensitivity: The child shows a reduced reaction to sensory stimulation and does not respond quickly enough. The gag, cough and swallow reflexes are not as active as they should be. The sensory threshold is elevated.

The following signs and symptoms may suggest that a child has abnormal sensory awareness: crying, withdrawal from food or drink, grimacing, blinking, an increase in tone, increase in involuntary movements, occurrence of spasms, and vomiting. A child who is *hypersensitive* may also gag excessively and be hypersensitive to touch in other parts of the body, such as the hands. The child who is *hyposensitive* will usually have an underactive gag reflex, a delayed or depressed swallow reflex, and a depressed or absent cough reflex. As a result of the underactivity of these protective responses, the hyposensitive child is at great risk of aspiration and its related health problems.

2. Oral stage

Once the child has taken food into his mouth, there are typical ways of controlling food and problems that can be recognised.

Jaw

Where there is a marked increase in tone, the jaw is often seen to be restricted in movement. It may be retracted (pulled back) and may open only a limited amount. Where postural tone is moderately increased, and in cases of fluctuating tone, the jaw is often seen to open and close too much. It lacks the stability that is needed for it to open with graded movement and to provide a basis for controlled selective movements of the tongue, lips and cheeks. The opening and closing of the jaw is often rhythmical, and there are no lateral or rotatory movements that would enable the child to chew. In some cases where children experience sharp increases in postural tone, or 'spasms', the jaw is clenched tightly shut in a 'bite reflex'.

This may be frightening and painful for the child as he is unable to release the bite. It is not uncommon for children to bite their own fingers or the inside of the mouth in this way.

Tongue

In cases of severe spasticity, the tongue may be lacking in movement and appear to be very 'bunched up' in the mouth. It may also be retracted. Where the increase in tone is more moderate, or where tone fluctuates, it is common to see the tongue moving only forward and backward in a kind of modified sucking pattern. This is usually in association with the opening and closing of the jaw. In cases where the child is quite extended, a tongue thrust may be seen. A child may cause an open sore to develop on the underside of his tongue due to persistent rubbing over the lower front teeth. Little or no movement of the tongue to the sides of the mouth is seen, except in some cases of children with involuntary movements.

Lips

The lips may remain inactive during eating, allowing considerable spillage (see section on the pre-oral stage). For this reason, it is common for children to be tipped back slightly in an attempt to keep food from falling or being pushed out of the mouth.

Throughout the oral stage, there is a risk of food being inhaled. It is important to listen to breathing sounds and to observe the child's facial expressions and postural tone carefully. Any possible indication of aspiration should be noted and monitored carefully.

3. Swallowing

The eating and drinking patterns described above often result in there being little opportunity for food to be mixed with saliva as a preparation for swallowing. When the child comes to swallow, food may therefore be inadequately prepared and difficult to swallow. Many children need to swallow many times to clear their mouths due to the inefficient movements of the tongue and lips. Food may be pushed forward out of the mouth through open lips, causing spillage.

In children who are hyposensitive inside their mouths, food may reach the back of the mouth without triggering off the swallow reflex (the swallow is 'delayed'). There is then a great danger of food entering the airway and causing coughing or choking. If the cough reflex is underactive, there may be 'silent aspiration'. This describes the situation where food goes into the airway without any obvious indication that this is happening.

Gastro-oesophageal reflux

As many as 75 per cent of children with cerebral palsy may suffer from the symptoms of gastro-oesophageal reflux (cited in Ravelli and Milla 1998). This is the regurgitation of food upwards from the stomach into the oesophagus. The primary cause is thought to be generalised dysmotility of the gut, caused by a dysfunction in the central nervous system and impaired function of the lower oesophageal sphincter. However, many other factors contribute to the occurrence of reflux in children with cerebral palsy, including habitual postures contributing to delayed gastric emptying, swallowing impairment resulting in poor clearance of acid from the oesophagus and constipation, and scoliosis or respiratory disease causing raised abdominal pressure (Sullivan 1997).

In some cases food may come up only a little way into the oesophagus, but in many cases refluxed food comes up to the opening of the airway where it can be vomited or aspirated, causing respiratory tract infections (Cass et al. 2005; Morton et al. 1999). Reflux may be the main cause of loss of appetite, food refusal, irritability during mealtimes and ill health. Serious malnourishment may result. This is because food coming up from the stomach is very acidic, and the high acidity may cause serious damage to the lining of the oesophagus (oesophagitis) and chronic pain associated with eating. Many cases of gastro-oesophageal reflux go unrecognised, or are misinterpreted as behavioural difficulty.

The child who suffers from this condition may appear to be hungry, but after a few mouthfuls becomes distressed and refuses to take more food. Turning away from food, arching the back and crying regularly at mealtimes is common. After mealtimes the child may appear to regurgitate small amounts of food for a long time, and to suffer badly from wind. Many such children vomit after eating. If gastro-oesophageal reflux is recognised, there is much that can be done to alleviate the problem by managing the texture of food that the child is given, and the position used for eating and drinking. Management by medication is becoming commonplace in some countries. In more severe cases, surgery (fundoplication) may be necessary (Sullivan 1997).

Communication at mealtimes

Assessment of mealtimes cannot be complete without an evaluation of the process of communication. From early infancy and throughout childhood, feeding times play an essential role in helping children to learn communication skills. In addition, good communication is essential for children to be able to eat in a safe and relaxed manner.

During a mealtime, it is important to observe the interaction between child and carer. How are likes and dislikes communicated? How does the carer know whether the child has had enough or wants more, or whether the eating process is causing discomfort? Many children with cerebral palsy who have eating and drinking problems also have significant communication difficulties and must attempt to communicate such messages via *non-verbal* means. These include facial expressions, eye movements, using the voice, gestures or whole body movements. With a little practice, an observer can begin to identify what a child is attempting to communicate. For example, a child who is looking at a drink is probably indicating thirst and asking for a drink. A child who is becoming unstable and turning away from food is probably communicating they don't want any more, or that they are in discomfort. Until such messages are understood by the person assisting in the eating and drinking process, and a means of resolving communication difficulties has been found, improvements in managing mealtimes and the safety of eating and drinking will only be limited.

MANAGEMENT OF EATING AND DRINKING DIFFICULTIES

The therapist's priority in managing eating and drinking problems should be to make the process of eating and drinking as safe as possible. The health of the child is of paramount importance, and therefore the prevention or minimisation of aspiration and gastro-oesophageal reflux, and provision of an adequate diet, should be immediate priorities. Most parents will be relieved to be able to describe their concerns about mealtimes and eating habits to a therapist. It is important to listen to these concerns and to work with the parent and child together to address them in practical ways.

The key to helping children who have difficulty in eating and drinking is understanding how the oral patterns arise from the child's overall patterns of movement. A young child whose jaw is open, who demonstrates a tongue thrust and minimal lip closure, for example, probably shows many other features of the pattern of extension. Effective management of eating difficulties is dependent on first establishing a stable position where tone is as normal as possible and the pattern of extension is minimised as described below. The following chart offers a broad guide to assist therapists in recognising how some eating and drinking characteristics relate to overall patterns of movement of extension and flexion.

	Extension	Flexion
Jaw	• Open jaw. Thrusting movement with little grading. Often retracted • Lower jaw may have an 'open bite', so that the front teeth are apart even when the mouth is closed	• Jaw closed. The range of movement is limited • Bite reflex may occur • Tooth grinding may also occur
Tongue	• May be 'bunched' (with very high tone). Usually tongue thrusting seen • Tongue may be retracted if the back of the neck is shortened	• May be bunched (with high tone) and elevated • Limited range of movement
Lips	• Often open at rest. May be retracted or pulled back. Sometimes quite immobile (when high tone)	• Often closed. Child may bite lips and cheeks causing pain and sores • Limited range of movement. Often pulled to one side with spasms
Swallow	• Difficult to initiate (often no lip closure) • Food may be pushed out by tongue • The swallow reflex may be delayed • High risk of aspiration	• Difficult to initiate due to limited tongue movement. Tongue movement is generally restricted

The ability to eat and drink safely may be greatly affected by the child's position at eating and drinking times. There is little benefit in changing the way in which children chew or drink, for example, without first ensuring that their posture and alignment are optimal. Although no two children are exactly alike, principles of safe positioning for eating and drinking can be identified. These principles can be applied whether a sitting or supported standing position is adopted for mealtimes.

General principles of positioning for eating and drinking

1. Stability
A good position for meal times requires the whole child to be well supported and in a stable position. Head and trunk stability are essential for safe eating. As food approaches, the child may become stiffer or experience more involuntary movements, but the position should allow the child to remain as still as possible. The child must feel comfortable, secure and relaxed.

2. Alignment and symmetry
The ability to control the mouth for eating and drinking is dependent on the head and trunk being not only stable but also in good alignment. The body should be as symmetrical as possible, with the head in midline and the trunk well aligned.

3. Elongation of the back of the neck
Regardless of whether we are eating in a sitting, standing or reclining position, we always maintain elongation of the back of our necks when we are eating and drinking, and keep our chin tucked in. This is the most important aspect of positioning, and one which should not be compromised.

When the head is in line with the trunk, and the back of the neck elongated, we can provide the maximum protection for our airways, to prevent food or liquid being aspirated. When we allow the head to tip back, there is an increased risk of choking or of food entering the airway. The spine should be straight. If the child's back is rounded in a sitting or standing position, the child will extend his neck, compromising the effective protection of his airway. If the feeder feels resistance to elongation of the back of the child's neck, then careful assessment of the spine will often reveal that it is flexed. Many children have a degree of long-term shortening of the back of the neck and flexion of the upper spine as a result of tone and position over a prolonged period. In these cases it is often helpful to allow the child to extend a little at the hips, which in turn will allow better extension of the spine and elongation of the back of the neck.

The majority of children with eating and drinking problems require assistance to achieve this position. It is therefore often helpful to use a handling technique known as *oral control* to keep the head and trunk stable and maintain elongation of the back of the neck.

4. Comfort

Children should be comfortable and as relaxed as possible during eating and drinking. This is so that their tone remains as stable as possible and their position generally still, allowing more normal patterns of movement. Anxiety about mealtimes often causes an increase in tone, involuntary movements or the occurrence of spasms, and this in turn makes the process of eating and drinking more difficult.

Some useful positions for meal times:

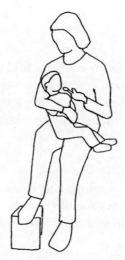

Figure 9.1
The feeder can use her leg to help keep the child's spine straight, and by sinking the child's hips down a little, can inhibit extension. Oral control may be provided as necessary

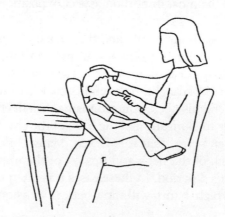

Figure 9.2
The feeder can keep the child's head position stable, and maintain face-to-face contact to facilitate communication. This position is more suitable for younger children

5. Position of the mealtime assistant

The position of the feeder in relation to the child who is eating has a significant effect on the child's own position, and therefore on her eating patterns. The children ideally should be able to look at the person who is feeding her, and this can be done in such a way as to encourage the optimum position of the head, keeping the back of the neck elongated and the chin tucked in. The child needs to be able to make eye contact with her feeder so that she can communicate her needs and feelings during the meal, and also be able to watch food coming towards her. In addition the feeder should be comfortable enough to maintain the feeding position throughout.

6. Supporting the feet

Ideally, a child's feet should be supported on the floor or a footrest to increase her stability. There are some children, however, who will use their feet to push against a flat surface, and this will make them unstable. In these cases it is better for the child's feet to be left unsupported.

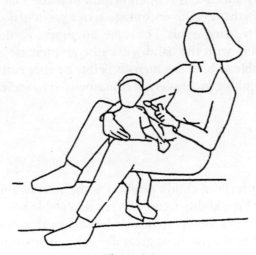

Figure 9.3
Sitting on a low bench. The child is well supported by the feeder's legs,
enabling one hand to provide oral control and the other to present food

Sitting, standing or reclining?

Whichever position a child is placed in to eat, whether on the lap or in a chair or other piece of equipment, the above principles can be used a guide. If a child is in a semi-reclined position on the lap, for example, it remains essential to ensure that the back of the neck is elongated and the chin tucked in. Figures 9.1, 9.2 and 9.3 show some useful positions to try with young children. In general it is easier to maintain a good position while feeding a young child on the lap. This is because the feeder can adjust position to give maximum support to the child. The position used should be dictated by what makes the child most easily obtain and maintain alignment to stay as safe as possible.

Involving the child's hands

From the earliest stages in feeding babies and young children, it is important to involve their hands. Hands play a vital role in giving children sensory input from which they can learn, and in enabling them to play an active part in controlling the eating and drinking process. Children as young as 4 months can use their hands to pull food towards their mouths or push it away. When feeding children with cerebral palsy, we can encourage them to place their hands around a bottle if one is used, or to feel the food with their fingers. It may be necessary to grade this stimulation very carefully so that the child's tone and movements are not negatively affected. It is often helpful to place a table or other flat surface in front of the child during the meal to encourage active participation both in exploration of the food and in communicating needs. For some, attempts to hold a bottle or spoon which involve the child grasping with the hand will cause an increase in tone. When this is the case, the child may be able to hold the utensils before or after eating, or in a play situation, so that the eating and drinking process is not compromised by increasing tone or involuntary movements.

Oral control

The most important aspect of a child's position is the relationship between the head and trunk. Head control, and the ability to use the jaw as a stable basis from which the tongue, lips and cheeks can work is a vital prerequisite for safe swallowing, chewing and drinking. Many children with cerebral palsy have great difficulty maintaining a stable head position themselves, and as a result they often have ungraded movements of the jaw.

When a child has poor head control or difficulty controlling their jaw movements, oral control may be provided by the person assisting. The mealtime assistant can use arm and hand to maintain a good head position, and to provide the stability upon which the child can move the jaw in a more controlled and graded way.

The assistant's arm is placed around the back of the child's neck. The upper part of the arm or inside of the elbow is used to maintain elongation of the back of the neck. The middle finger is placed under the chin, just behind the bone and applies firm pressure to keep the jaw stable. As the child opens their mouth, the finger maintains constant pressure, allowing just sufficient opening for the food to be placed in the child's mouth, and then helping the child to maintain a closed mouth during swallowing.

The index finger is usually placed on the front of the child's chin, just below the lip. This helps to keep the head position stable, and to counter the upward pressure from the middle finger under the chin (thus ensuring that the head is not tipped upwards). When the jaw is stable, the lower lip will usually be able to function well, but in cases where it does not, the feeder's index finger can be used to guide it to close when appropriate.

The feeder's thumb rests on the child's face near the ear, or is held right away from the face. It's role is mainly to help the feeder keep their hand in a stable position, although rarely it may help to prevent the jaw from deviating to one side or the other. Occasionally the thumb may interfere with the eating process due to a retained rooting reflex which causes the child to turn towards it. In these cases it will help to make sure there is no contact between the thumb and the side of the face.

It may take a little while for some children to feel comfortable with oral control. For most children it is best to introduce it at a snack time rather than at a main meal. The handling should be firm and consistent, so that the child does not feel the hand moving around. It may be helpful to apply oral control at first with the thumb only, stabilising the jaw from below, with the rest of the fingers placed on the sternum. The sternum is then used as a key point of control, and can help to prevent the child from pushing back into extension.

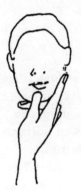

Figure 9.4a
Oral control: provided by someone sitting in front of the child

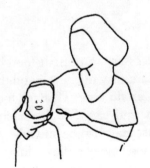

Figure 9.4b
Oral control: provided from the side

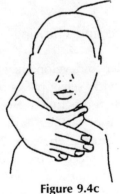

Figure 9.4c
Oral control: from the side, using the sternum as key point of control. This often works well when assisting a young child on the lap or when sitting on a bench as shown before

Spoon-feeding

Use oral control to keep the head in a good position and to maintain stability of the jaw. Ideally, the spoon should have a flat bowl, enabling the child to feel the food on his lips when they close, and to effectively remove it. It may be helpful to use a durable plastic spoon so that the child is not afraid of biting on hard metal.

Food presented by spoon should be of a uniform 'mashed' consistency. Try to avoid very runny textures or food containing hard lumps. If the food is hard enough to need chewing it is better to give it by hand as described below.

Always present the spoon in the midline, and place it flat on the front of the tongue. Provision of oral control enables the jaw to open just enough to allow the spoon into the mouth. Apply firm pressure downward on the front of the tongue, and then wait for the child to begin to lower the top lip. As they do so, you may assist by closing the lower jaw, and removing the spoon. This is done in one smooth movement, so that there is only one opening and closure of the jaw, and the child does not have the opportunity to bite up and down on the spoon. Maintain oral closure until that mouthful has been completely swallowed and you have a heard a clear breath. You can then proceed with the next spoonful.

The application of firm downward pressure on the front of the tongue helps to bring the tongue to a normal starting point from which to swallow, and to inhibit tongue thrusting. Make sure that the spoon does not press backward on the tongue, since this may cause the child to gag. The downward pressure from the spoon also facilitates lip closure and enables the child to remove food from the spoon without it being scraped off against the top teeth.

Developing chewing

In order to develop chewing, it is necessary to present food by hand or finger feeding. To begin with, select pieces of food that are easy to chew. Food that dissolves or becomes very soft when it is first chewed is ideal. Certain types of snack food such Quavers and Wotsits dissolve once they have been bitten, and can then be safely swallowed without fear of pieces causing choking. Pieces of toast may also be suitable, or French fries.

Place a piece of 'bite and dissolve' food between the child's teeth on the side of the mouth, coming from the midline, and hold it there. Use oral control to ensure that the head is kept in a good position, and that the mouth opens and closes with graded movement. The child may bite on the food straight away, but if he does not, then move the food slightly to stimulate biting. As the child opens and closes his jaw to chew, it is usually possible to see that lateral movement of the tongue is also stimulated. Keep holding the food at the side of the child's mouth until it is softened and then sucked onto the tongue. It will then be further sucked and then swallowed. Use oral control throughout to ensure lip closure during swallowing and to maintain graded jaw movements.

The role of the oral control is to maintain alignment and limit jaw opening. It is not to move the jaw in a chewing pattern. The child will move his jaw himself, and the hand providing oral control acts as a limiter, to keep this movement within a normal range.

As the child becomes accustomed to chewing foods that dissolve easily, progress to foods that are more chewable: bread, cooked vegetables and ripe fruit can all be given by being placed to the sides of the mouth. Avoid hard foods such as raw carrot and apple, which may be dangerous and cause choking. Try to finger-feed some food at each mealtime. Some children may take food more easily in this way than from a spoon. It is also important for the child to be able to feel the texture of the food in his hands. Ideally, every texture should be introduced to the hands prior to being placed in the mouth, although the child may not be able to hold the food and eat at the same time.

For many children with cerebral palsy, food that needs to be chewed will always have to be presented in this way. Some children will progress to being able to move food to the sides of their mouths themselves, and then may be able to finger-feed themselves. Those children who have very poor head and jaw control may benefit from practising chewing in safety by being given the opportunity to chew on some dried fruit wrapped in a pouch made of a cotton handkerchief or piece of muslin which is held by the feeder and placed between the teeth to the side of the mouth. In this way, the child can taste the dried fruit and practise the movements of chewing without danger of choking.

Drinking

To develop a safe drinking pattern, good positioning and use of oral control is very important. Many children find it difficult to control thin, runny fluids in their mouths, and are therefore in danger of frequent choking during drinking. For this reason it is often best to introduce drinking with liquids that are naturally thick, such as puréed fruit, yoghurt, custard or drinks thickened by mixing in a thickening agent. Thick fluids move slowly and are relatively heavy, thereby giving increased sensory information to the mouth. Introduce the thickened liquids in an open cup. A soft plastic cup with a 'cut-out' may be useful so that the child does not need to tip their head back as the cup is tipped up. A Doidy cup (which slopes to one side) is another suitable alternative which enables the cup to be tipped while the child's head stays upright.

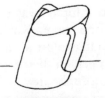

Figure 9.5
A Doidy cup

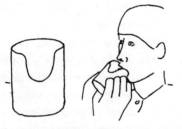

Figure 9.6
A cup with a small piece cut out to enable the cup to be tipped without the child's neck extending

Use oral control. Tip the cup before presenting it to the child so that the fluid is already at the rim. Place the cup on the lower lip in front of the teeth. Tip so that the liquid is even in the mouth, and wait for the child to move their top lip. The child will be able to feel the liquid on the lips since the mouth is only slightly open.

Young children often learn to drink from a cup with a spout. This is not appropriate for children with cerebral palsy since use of a spout reinforces an immature sucking pattern, and may cause exaggerated tongue thrusting to develop.

Once the child has got used to taking a few sips in this way, try to establish a rhythm of drinking. In this way he can anticipate that he will do three sips, for example, and then the cup will be removed for him to close his lips to swallow and then breath comfortably. It may be helpful to count aloud—one, two, three, rest. The child may tolerate more sips, but the feeder should ensure that the child's pattern of breathing is not compromised and there is no risk of aspiration.

SOME SPECIFIC PROBLEMS

1. Managing problems of sensation

On the basis of an initial assessment it is often difficult to evaluate the nature and extent of sensory problems. The superficial symptoms of hypersensitivity and hyposensitivity may appear similar; in both cases, the child may dislike eating and drinking and may turn away from food. In many cases, children who are hyposensitive intra-orally may also be hyper-sensitive on the face and around the mouth in particular.

When managing a child with sensory problems the priority is to ensure that his airway is adequately protected during eating and drinking. Through careful manipulation of the child's position, texture of food and fluids, and use of feeding techniques, it is usually possible to bring about a significant change in eating patterns and minimise health risks. Management comprises a combination of grading the sensory stimulation of eating so that the child can swallow most effectively, and, through use of handling techniques and good positioning, enabling the child to grade his motor responses during eating, which in turn reinforces more normal sensation.

The child who is *hypersensitive* will benefit from therapeutic input away from mealtimes. Introduce the child to things such as a toothbrush, a rattle or a spoon, which can be safely explored by putting them in the mouth. Encourage the child to explore a variety of textures in this way. Young children enjoy playing with their own fingers in their mouths, and may gradually get used to playing with a small toothbrush or soft rubber toy.

By progressing in very small steps, expect the child to tolerate exploring things in the mouth for slightly longer periods, and introduce a few different textures. When the child expresses slight anxiety or discomfort at the toy, keep still and wait for the child to adjust to the stimulation and relax. It is important not to push the child beyond what can be comfortably tolerated. If the experience becomes unpleasant or over-stimulating, then increased hypersensitivity and hypertonicity will result, rather than an ability to tolerate stimulation at a more normal level. Remember that the goal of this process is to enable the child to cope better with a variety of textures of food, and to be able to eat and drink more safely.

The child who is *hyposensitive* often responds more effectively to the stimulation of food and drink in his mouth when given adequate time. Good positioning and oral control is essential to ensure protection of the airway. Careful spoon-feeding of food of a cohesive, mashed texture, with firm pressure applied onto the tongue to facilitate good tongue movement, can often stimulate a safe swallow. Food that is cold, or that has a strong flavour (spicy food) may be easier for the child to eat. When given ample time and adequate stimulation, depressed reflexes can improve. Always ensure a child has time to clear each mouthful and breathe comfortably between each mouthful. Runny fluid may be easily aspirated in the hyposensitive child, and is often best substituted by thickened liquids.

2. Tongue thrust

A tongue thrust is a forward–backward sucking movement which may be exaggerated by increased tone. It is part of an extensor pattern and is indicative of a lack of jaw stability. The child with a tongue thrust usually has little or no spontaneous lateral movement of the tongue, or ability to chew.

A tongue thrust can usually be modified or inhibited by careful positioning and use of oral control. The use of a good spoon-feeding technique is another effective way of inhibiting tongue thrust and facilitating more normal tongue movement patterns. Presentation of runny food on a spoon often exaggerates tongue thrusting and therefore should be avoided. Food of a more cohesive, mashed texture is suitable for spoon-feeding. Work towards developing chewing, and thereby a more normal range of tongue movements; and drinking, with provision of oral control aimed at controlling fluid intake from an open cup.

3. Tonic bite reflex

This is an often distressing pattern of biting that occurs without voluntary control by the child. It involves a sudden increase in tone accompanied by sustained biting together of the jaws and is usually triggered by touch, especially to the front teeth. The tonic bite reflex is almost always part of a generalised flexor spasm and should not be seen as something that involves the mouth in isolation. It is usually indicative of some degree of hypersensitivity, and occurs in children whose tone can rise sharply to quite high levels of spasticity. Children with bite reflexes may also grind their teeth and accidentally bite their own cheeks, tongue or fingers.

Reducing hypersensitivity is a vital part of helping a child to overcome a bite reflex. Play which involves the child in handling a variety of textures and getting used to releasing grasp is important. Positioning to minimise the occurrence of flexor spasms should be considered; children with bite reflexes may be able to eat and drink with less disturbance from spasms in a prone standing frame, with the provision of good oral control. It may, of course, take some preparation to enable a child to stand comfortably in a standing frame before being able to eat or drink in this position. Development of chewing will lead to a more normal set of movement patterns of the jaw and tongue; chewing at the beginning of a meal may help to relax the jaw. Spoon-feeding is often difficult in children with strong bite reflexes, but use of a good technique, which will at first trigger the bite reflex to occur, can be very effective in diminishing the occurrence of the bite. Children who have strong bite reflexes often associate eating and drinking with pain and fear. It is important for the mealtime assistant to remain calm when the bite reflex occurs, to encourage the child to remain as relaxed as possible and to wait for the spasm to pass. Anxiety in this situation invariably causes tone to increase further and thereby exacerbates the problem.

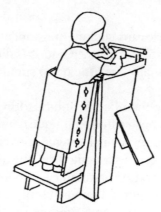

Figure 9.7
Child in prone standing frame. This position is often helpful for children
who have tonic bite reflexes or who suffer from gastro-oesophageal reflux

4. Gastro-oesophageal reflux

Children who suffer from gastro-oesophageal reflux can be helped by careful positioning during and after mealtimes, by controlling the texture of food, and by the timing of mealtimes and snacks. Gastro-oesophageal reflux may be exacerbated by an increase in abdominal pressure, and for many children this can be minimised by careful positioning. Positioning in a prone standing frame, for example, will minimise the effects of flexor spasms and keep the child in a position where gravity helps the passage of food through the digestive system, and in particular through the stomach. Many children will be helped by remaining in an upright or extended position after eating, for up to half an hour or longer if possible. For a child who cannot be stood in this way, discomfort associated with gastro-oesophageal reflux may be relieved by holding her in an extended position, while keeping her head elevated as shown. In this position, gastric emptying is aided and flexor spasms may be inhibited. Children may also benefit from sleeping with their mattress tilted up to 30 degrees, so that gravity aids the passage of food through the digestive system. (This can most easily be done by elevating the head end of the bed.)

Children may be less prone to gastro-oesophageal reflux if they do not eat big quantities of food at any one time. The occurrence of reflux may be reduced by offering four or five smaller meals each day, rather than three large ones. In this way, the stomach does not become full and distended, and gastro-oesophageal reflux is less likely to occur.

Introduction of thick liquids for drinking may be helpful, since food of a thicker texture is less likely to be refluxed than runny liquids. From 4 months old, children can be introduced to solid food. In many cases a reduction in the incidence of vomiting and reflux occurs at this stage.

Children who suffer from oesophagitis often find acidic foods such as fruit painful to swallow. Avoidance of very acidic food may help to maintain an adequate diet in children who may potentially refuse to eat.

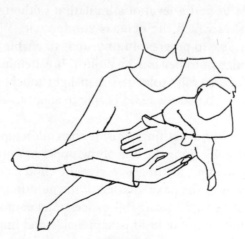

Figure 9.8
Carrying position for inhibition of flexor spasms and relief of discomfort associated with gastro-oesophageal reflux. Gravity aids gastric emptying and abdominal pressure is kept as stable as possible

THE IMPORTANCE OF ORAL HYGIENE

Children with cerebral palsy are particularly susceptible to dental caries and gum disease, which could lead to discomfort in the mouth and exacerbation of eating and drinking problems. This is due in part to limited selective tongue movements which normally help to keep teeth clean, lack of saliva due to dribbling, hypersensitivity, and diets which may be high in sugar to maximise calorie intake. Tooth and gum problems often make it hard for children to tolerate having their teeth cleaned. Good dental hygiene should be introduced from a very young age to minimise the occurrence of dental health problems. Provision of healthy oral stimulation can help to increase tolerance of food textures and lay a good foundation for the development of chewing and saliva control (Winstock 1994 and forthcoming).

Gum massage

Even before an infant's first teeth have erupted, regular gum massage can be provided. It is important that the child is comfortable with this, that she can safely swallow the increase in saliva caused by the stimulation, and that she is positioned with her head upright, chin tucked in and back of the neck elongated. For many children, the provision of oral control is necessary to maintain such a stable position, as in feeding.

Gum massage should be pleasurable for a child, and if gagging is caused or the child shows any sign of distress, it should be brought to a level that the child can comfortably tolerate. It is always possible to find a level of stimulation (although this may be very low indeed for some children) at which the child is comfortable. When this level has been found, the carer should be able to progress in tiny steps to enable the child to comfortably tolerate a little more stimulation to her face or mouth. It is helpful to remember that firm, steady pressure is always more easily tolerated than light touch, and that all movements should be slow and rhythmic so that the child is able to adapt to every movement she feels and remain relaxed.

The carer may start by rolling a wet finger inside the child's top lip, slightly to one side. Gradually rub the finger steadily along the line of the upper jaw on one side, backward and forward a couple of times. Remove the finger to give the child a chance to swallow and remain relaxed, then proceed with the next 'quarter' of the mouth. Finally, massage along the child's lower gums in the same way. During this process oral control will be necessary for a majority of children to ensure that the head is kept stable and that the child does not gag. Oral control will also enable the carer to keep the mouth as closed as possible during this process. It may be advisable to wear protective rubber gloves for this procedure to minimise the possibility of transfer of infection between the carer and child.

Tooth brushing

Once the child starts to develop teeth, this process can be carried out with a small toothbrush. If a baby's rubber toothbrush is available, many young children will enjoy munching on this. It may also provide good practice for developing chewing skills. If the child finds it too difficult to tolerate a toothbrush, then it is preferable to continue tooth cleaning with a finger, and with the possible introduction of a small amount of toothpaste.

The toothbrush is used in a similar pattern to the finger in gum massage. Oral control is usually necessary to ensure that the child's head is held in a stable upright position, maintaining elongation of the back of the neck. Treat the mouth in four sections. When brushing the upper jaw, brush the teeth from top to bottom, and from the back of the mouth to the front. When brushing the lower jaw, brush the teeth from bottom to top, and again, from the back of the mouth to the front. After each section remove the brush, allowing the child enough time to spit out any excess water or toothpaste, and to do several relaxed breaths before beginning the next section. Tooth brushing is a very stimulatory activity, and most children will need time to get used to it. It should not cause gagging, and if it appears to be doing so, then it is wise to use a finger instead of the brush for a while. It may also be advisable to bring the child into a more prone position where gravity aids saliva to drain forward rather than back into the pharynx.

Nutritional issues

Many children with eating and drinking difficulties do not receive an adequate diet. It is common for children with cerebral palsy to suffer from constipation and to be short, have low muscle bulk and be underweight for their age (Reilly et al. 1996).

To some extent, poor growth may be minimised by providing as many calories as possible in the texture that the child can eat the most efficiently. For example, some children are able to drink thickened liquids from a cup more easily than they can take solid foods in other forms. In these cases it would be beneficial to provide as many calories in a liquid texture as possible.

Poor fluid intake often contributes to the tendency of many children with cerebral palsy to be constipated. Increasing fluid intake often requires development of drinking skills as outlined earlier, and the introduction of drinking thickened liquids. It is particularly important to try to increase the amount of water intake in cases of constipation.

Looking after a child with eating and drinking difficulties may cause considerable stress and anxiety to carers. In many instances, carers spend excessive amounts of time trying to give sufficient food to the children in their care. It may often be found that after

30–40 minutes of eating and drinking, children become so fatigued that beyond this time negligible amounts of food are consumed. For many children, it is advisable to take a break from the meal at this point, and to consider introducing an additional snack to the daily routine to provide further nutrition. In this way, an overall reduction in the feeding time can be made without reducing the quantity of food or fluid that is consumed. Where the advice of a dietician is available it can be extremely beneficial.

In some cases, a baby or child may experience such difficulty in eating or drinking that she does not take in adequate nourishment. Where this is the case in the Western world feeding of a specially prepared meal via a *naso-gastric tube* or a *gastrostomy tube* is recommended. A naso-gastric tube can itself exacerbate some eating and drinking problems since it interferes with the normal eating and drinking process, but a gastrostomy tube, although it requires insertion by a surgeon in a hospital setting, still allows the child the possibility of eating comfortably, and does not impose the pressure of needing to meet all the child's nutritional needs in this way (Sullivan et al. 2004).

The decision to implement the use of gastrostomy feeding is one that is usually taken by a team which includes a speech and language therapist and a paediatrician. Sullivan et al. (2005) studied 57 children who had gastrostomies placed, aged between 5 months and 17 years of age. Almost all the parents reported a significant improvement in their child's health after the intervention and a significant reduction in time spent feeding. The children gained weight and serious complications were only 'rare'. An earlier study also demonstrated clear and measurable improvements in the quality of life of carers after insertion of a gastrostomy tube (Sullivan et al. 2004).

REFERENCES

Cass, H., C. Wallis, H. Ryan, S. Reilly and K. McHugh. 2005. 'Assessing Pulmonary Consequences of Dysphagia in Children with Neurological Disabilities: When to Intervene?', *Developmental Medicine and Child Neurology* 47: 347–52.

Evans Morris, S. and M. Dunn Klein. 2000. *Pre-Feeding Skills: A Comprehensive Resource for Mealtime Development*, 2nd edition Tucson, AZ: Therapy Skill Builders.

Gisel, E.G. and J. Patrick. 1988. 'Identification of Children with Cerebral Palsy, Unable to Maintain a Normal Nutritional State', *Lancet* 1: 283–86.

Gisel, E.G., T. Applegate-Ferrante, J. Benson and J.F. Bosma. 1996. 'Oral-Motor Skills Following Sensorimotor Therapy in Two Groups of Moderately Dysphagic Children with Cerebral Palsy: Aspiration vs Nonaspiration', *Dysphagia* 11: 59–71.

Humphrey, T. 1970. 'Reflex Activity in the Oral and Facial Area of the Human Fetus', in J.F. Bosma, ed., *Second Symposium on Oral Sensation and Perception*, pp. 195–233. Springfield, IL: Thomas.

Larnert, G. and O. Ekberg. 1995. 'Positioning Improves the Oral and Pharyngeal Swallowing Function in Children with Cerebral Palsy', *Acta Paediatrica* 84: 689–92.

Morton, R.E., R. Wheatley and J. Minford. 1999. 'Respiratory Tract Infections due to Direct and Reflux Aspiration in Children with Severe Neurodisability', *Developmental Medicine and Child Neurology* 41: 329–34.

Ravelli, A.M. and P. Milla. 1998. 'Vomiting and Gastroesophageal Motor Activity in Children with Disorders of the Central Nervous System', *Journal of Pediatric Gastroenterology and Nutrition* 26: 56–63.

Reilly, S., D. Skuse and X. Poblete. 1996. 'Prevalence of Feeding Problems and Oral Motor Dysfunction in Children with Cerebral Palsy: A Community Survey', *J Paediatrica* 129: 877–82.

Rempel, G.R., S.O. Colwell and R.P. Nelson. 1988. 'Growth in Children with Cerebral Palsy Fed via Gastrostomy', *Paediatrics* 82: 857–62.

Reyas, A.L., A.J. Cash, S.H. Green and I.W. Booth. 1993. 'Gastro-Oesophageal Reflux in Children with Cerebral Palsy', *Child Care Health and Development* 19: 109–18.

Sullivan, P. 1997. 'Gastrointestinal Problems in the Neurologically Impaired Child', *Balliere's Clinical Gastroenterology* 11(3), September.

Sullivan, P., E. Juszczak, A. Bachlet, B. Lambert, A. Vernon-Roberts, H. Grant, M. Eltumi, L. McLean, N. Alder and A. Thomas. 2005. 'Gastrostomy Tube Feeding in Children with Cerebral Palsy: A Prospepctive, Longitudinal Study', *Developmental Medicine and Child Neurology* 47(2): 77–85.

Sullivan, P., E. Juszczak, A. Bachlet, A. Thomas, B. Lambert, A. Vernon-Roberts, H. Grant, M. Eltumi, N. Alder and C. Jenkinson. 2004. 'Impact of Gastrostomy Tube Feeding on the Quality of Life of Carers of Children with Cerebral Palsy', *Developmental Medicine and Child Neurology* 46(12): 796–800.

Winstock, A. 1994 and forthcoming. *The Practical Management of Eating and Drinking Diffifculties in Children.* Bicester, UK: Winslow Press.

MARIAN BROWNE graduated from Sheffield University in 1986 with a Bachelor of Medical Science in Speech Science. She has worked as a Speech and Language Therapy Tutor at the Bobath Centre for Children with Cerebral Palsy, London, for 11 years and has also worked in the field of paediatrics in Cambridge and London. Marian has a particular interest in the management of eating and drinking difficulties and is involved in the postgraduate training of therapists in this field, in addition to working in private practice.

Appendix A

How to make equipment from appropriate paper-based technology (APT)

JEAN WESTMACOTT

APPROPRIATE paper-based technology (APT) is a cost-effective way to produce personally designed furniture or other objects for use and creativity from recycled paper and cardboard. It involves using flour and water paste to stick layers of corrugated cardboard together to make flat boards. At first they are soft, but once dry become relatively hard. While the stuck layers are drying they need to be pressed under a flat surface. The flat pieces for the item to be made are measured and cut from the dry board. The pieces will not be strong enough to bear someone's weight at this stage. They need reinforcement. This is done using techniques based on engineering principles to make the cardboard able to cope with the pressure and tension of use. Techniques include using layers of pasted paper, strengthening supports, tension rods and reinforced joints.

Materials needed

- **Paper**
- **Corrugated cardboard**
- **Thin cardboard for rods**
- **Flour for making paste**

Tools needed

- **Knives—one with a strong blade for cutting straight edges and one with a thin blade and sharp point for cutting holes. Kitchen knives work well**
- **Kettle or means for boiling water to make paste**
- **Bowl or jug and large spoon for making paste**

MAKING A CHAIR

These instructions are for a simple chair that lends itself to being adapted. You can make this chair with a curved back, sloping seat or knee-blocks. However, start with a simple version to practice. Your techniques are vitally important, as the weak materials you are using need care and attention to turn them into a strong weight-bearing chair.

Most of the techniques for any APT work are used in making this chair. They are explained in the instructions, and include:

- Steps for making paste
- Alternate layering for boards
- Pressing
- Rolling card into a rod
- Making straps
- Making 'angle irons' using thin card
- Strapping

Measuring

When measuring for a piece of furniture, such as a chair, use flat boards or books. It helps to remember that you are measuring for a chair, not around the curves of the body.

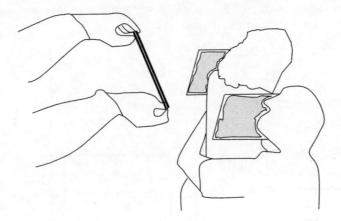

Measure the width of the child at shoulder height using two flat boards
(hold them parallel to each other)

Measurements needed	Examples from a 3-year-old, in centimetres
1. Seat height: From base of foot to top of flat surface where child is sitting	22
2. Seat depth: From behind knee to flat surface held behind child (at 90° angle to seat)	23
3. Height of backrest: From top of seat to flat surface held on shoulder (length of back)	30
4. Headrest (only if necessary): From below flat surface on shoulder to sufficient support point on head	15
5. Headrest (only if necessary): Width of head	

(continued)

(continued)

Measurements needed	Examples from a 3-year-old, in centimetres
6. Width of backrest: Between parallel flat surfaces held against arms (see illustration), i.e., width of shoulders	25
7. Seat width: Between parallel flat surfaces held against sides of hips, i.e., width of hips	22
8. Height of arm rest: From seat to elbow	
9. Height for table or tray: Optimal height from seat; check while the child is working, e.g., trying to write	14
10. Footrest (only if needed): Length of foot	15

Step-by-step chair instructions

1.

Start by making a sketch of the pieces you will need, along with their measurements. It can be a chair for yourself or for a child you have measured.

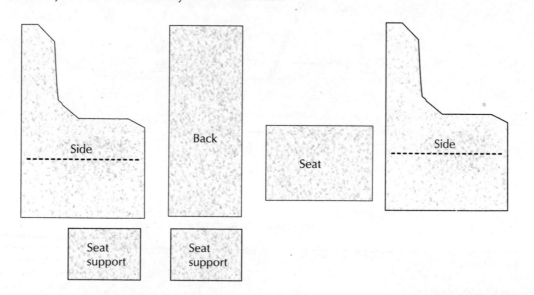

2.

Make paste. You will need two full tablespoons of flour. Flour can be wheat, *maida*, finely ground maize or cassava flour. Mix with about 100 ml of *cold* water until free of lumps, like smooth cream. Add about 400 ml (two cupfuls) of *rapidly boiling* water quickly, while continuing to stir.

MAKING PASTE

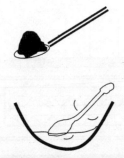 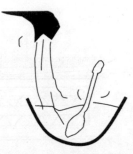

Mix two tablespoons of flour with
cold water—it should look like thick cream

Pour in water that is *still boiling*. Do this rapidly
while stirring. Pour in to make about 500 ml

The resultant paste should feel sticky.

3.

Make a large board (or two), big enough so the sides, seat, seat supports and back can be cut from it.
Layers can be made up of smaller pieces if you do not have large enough sizes. The number of layers
depends on the thickness of the cardboard and the size of the person using the stool, but do have
enough layers stacked so that the thickness of each board comes to about 2 cm. The boards will be
stronger if the corrugations of each layer run across the width and the length alternately.

Organise the layers for each board. Rub a thin layer of paste on *each* surface of the layers where
they will attach to each other.

ALTERNATE LAYERING FOR BOARDS

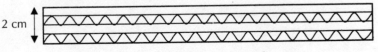

2 cm

Corrugations in alternate directions—edge view

4.

As soon as the pieces of cardboard are stuck together, they must be compressed. Place some sheets of
dry newspaper under the layered pieces with some more dry newspaper on top. Finally, place a flat
wooden board or table upside-down on this, making sure it covers the whole piece. This ensures
that the pasted layers will stick together evenly and dry *flat*. If necessary, put something to act as a
weight on top of the flat wooden board. Some books or a few bricks are sufficient.

5.

Open up and check and air out the layered pieces and change the newspaper every day until flat and
dry. This can take a few days even in dry weather.

6.

When the board is flat and dry it is time to draw out the pieces for the chair on the board. Start by
making sure one edge is totally straight by checking it with a long ruler made of the machine-cut

PRESSING

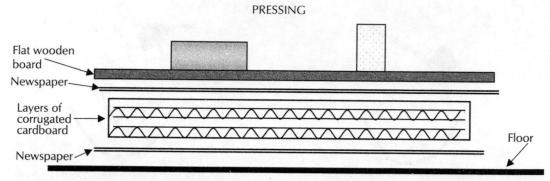

Dry sheets of newspaper on each side of boards being compressed under a flat wooden board

straight edge of a piece of cardboard. You may need to cut the layered board to make the edge straight. This is now the edge for the bottom of the chair.

7.

Cut two sides with the straight edge at the bottom to make sure the chair will not wobble.

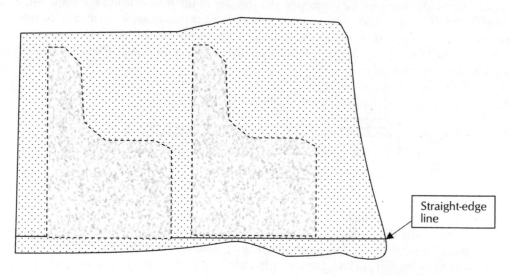

8.

Measure the width for your back, seat and seat supports (all these are the same width) and cut a long 'plank' of this width.

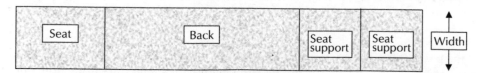

9.

Check that the width is the same for the back, seat and two seat supports.

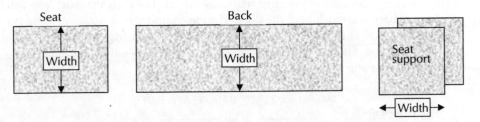

10.

Paste one seat support on the base of the back and press under a book or flat piece of wood. This will act as support for the back of the seat.

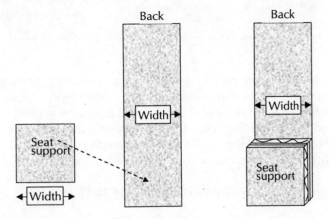

11.

One seat support is pasted onto the back of the chair and the other will be pasted and strapped further forward under the seat. Two rods will be made and used to tension the chair and help support the child's weight. This will be shown further on in these instructions. The second seat support is to be fixed just behind the rod that is under the seat near the front.

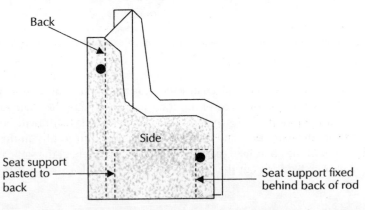

12.

Now make two rods from thin card. These must be 8 cm longer than the width of the chair. About 2 cm will stick out on either side of the chair when assembled. The ends that stick out will be split so they can be bent back and stuck onto the sides. The most important function of these two rods is to pull the sides together. They will strengthen the chair against moving and pulling *tension* forces when the chair is in use. The rods will take the strain. As well as tensioning, one rod will help support the seat and the other will support the back.

MEASURING THE CARD FOR A ROD

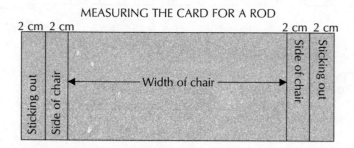

13.

Check in which direction the grain goes, by gently bending or rolling the card in each direction. The direction in which it bends most easily is where the grain runs. Rub paste all over the card. Roll it around a smooth broomstick handle or equivalent, so the grain goes along the length of the rod (so that it rolls easily and also because the rod will be stronger with the grain along its length). Pull it off the broomstick and leave to dry. If the outside edge threatens to pull away, make a small strap to hold them down strongly (see strapping instructions). Use the broomstick to make the next rod.

ROLLING CARD INTO A ROD

Roll tightly so there are no air gaps—the tighter the roll, the stronger the rod

14.

One rod will be placed directly behind the chair back near the top, the other under the seat in front of the seat support. Draw lines on one side of the chair to mark where the chair back will be and to mark the level of the seat. Mark the holes for the two supporting rods by drawing around the ends of the rods, in order to get the exact size and to make sure they will fit tightly in the holes. Cut these holes with the two sides of the chair held together so that the holes are at the same place in each side. Use a knife with a narrow blade to cut the curved edges for the holes.

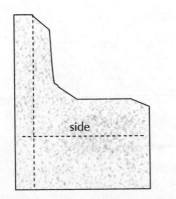
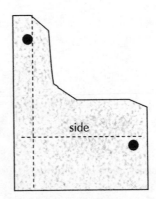

15.
Fit all the pieces together. Trim edges with a knife, if necessary, until everything fits well.

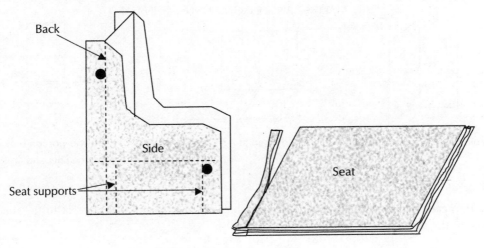

When every part fits together satisfactorily, it is time to paste.

16.
Rub paste on all the edges and surfaces that will be attached to others. Use a strip of cloth or piece of string to tie around the sides of the chair temporarily so that the seat and back are held together and kept steady. Paste up some paper to make straps.

17.
Start with the joints and make 'angle irons' from thin card.

18.
Make two angle irons. Rub paste on both sides and rub the angle irons into the back corners under the seat of the chair. This helps the three sides to connect—but they now need strapping. Place and rub the straps over the angle irons. This may require a little more paste.

MAKING STRAPS

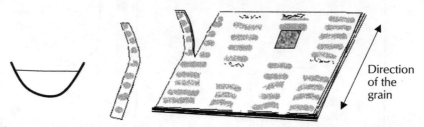

Direction of the grain

Rub paste thinly over a piece of newspaper. Place another piece of the same size on top, making sure the grain of the paper is running in the same direction (the grain runs in the direction in which the paper tears easily). Add at least four layers of paper so that when you tear off a narrow strap of layered paper it will be strong enough not to break when you pull it holding onto each end of the strap. Always tear, rather than cut, the paper as a rough edge sticks better than a cut edge. It is also quicker to tear than cut!

MAKING 'ANGLE IRONS' USING THIN CARD

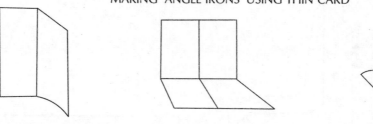

Fold piece of card in half   Fold again at right angles   Tear lower portion only in half, along the line, and cross over

19.

Use thin card folded in half to make small angle irons to help connect the seat to the sides. Place them on the underside of the seat close to the front.

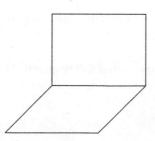

20.

Fix the other seat support just behind the rod, using straps. Attach the seat to the sides of the chair with angle irons.

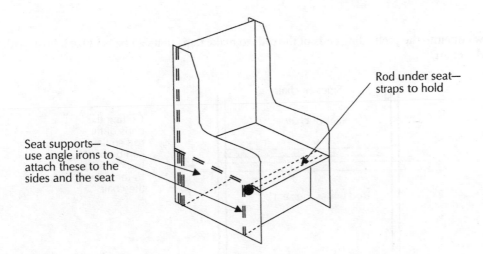

Rod under seat—
straps to hold

Seat supports—
use angle irons to
attach these to the
sides and the seat

21.
Strap over all these joints. Use straps of layered paper. These can overlap each other. Each strap should be only about 3 cm wide. (When covering edges that are curved this should be far narrower.) Turn the chair upside-down and support it on some bricks to make strapping under the seat easier. Stick straps over the rod and rub to make a tight connection between the rod and seat.

STRAPPING

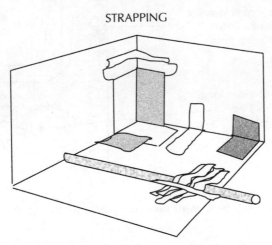

Strong joints make the chair strong

22.
Once the inner joints are securely strapped, the strip of cloth or piece of string can be removed before strapping all the joints on the outside of the chair.

23.

Now saw cuts into the protruding ends of the rods to make flaps that can be bent back flush with the side of the chair.

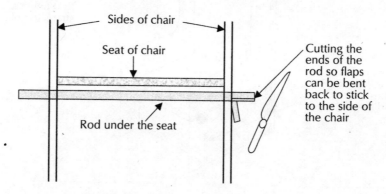

Sides of chair

Seat of chair

Cutting the ends of the rod so flaps can be bent back to stick to the side of the chair

Rod under the seat

24.

Bend the cut ends of the rods back and rub to flatten them against the sides of the chair. Then paste and stick back using straps.

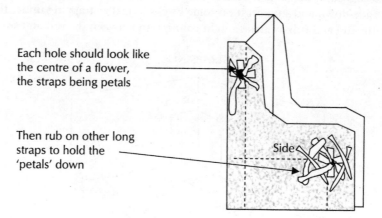

Each hole should look like the centre of a flower, the straps being petals

Then rub on other long straps to hold the 'petals' down

Side

25.

Check that it is all rubbed down well, with no small pieces lifting up or air bubbles between the layers.

26.

Then place and rub straps across all the edges to make them neat and strong.

27.

When the joints and edges are completely strapped, the remaining surfaces can be filled more quickly. Use mosaics of pasted paper, each one torn no larger than 7 × 7 cm, so that they do not wrinkle.

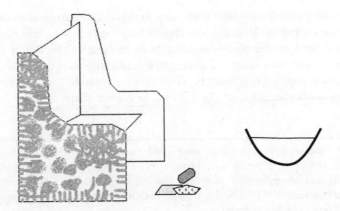

28.
Leave the chair until it is 100 per cent dry and hard. In dry weather this only takes a week. Keep turning it so the inside is exposed to the air for drying as well as the outside.

29.
Then there is the fun of adding a decorative finish. The chair can be decorated with a single layer of gift paper, brown paper or a collage of pictures from magazines. Once dry, clear varnish can be used to give a professional finish and make the chair splash-proof.

30.
Alternatively, gloss paint or wood paint can be used (it will block out the newspaper print).

Making a chair with a curved back

Once you have mastered the techniques you can make all sort of chairs. The chair illustrated below has a sloping back that is curved, and a seat that slopes down. For this design you need to make the

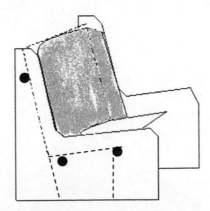

sides slightly longer so the back can slope with support. Make one extra rod to support the seat (the dotted lines show the supports). To make this chair with a curved back, first make the chair with a flat back, then paste on a curved piece (measure from the seat to the top of the back to get the length). This is made from two layers of corrugated cardboard pasted together, with both layers having the corrugations running downwards. This makes it possible to create a curve. Strap this on while it is still damp with paste so it will be held in the correct shape to dry.

JEAN WESTMACOTT has worked in this field since 1980. In 1988 the UK's Overseas Development Agency funded her training in APT by Bevill Packer in Zimbabwe. Since then she has researched and trained extensively in the methods, safety and design of APT furniture. She has taught on the Community Disabilities Studies course at the Centre of International Child Health, University College London, and provided training for Voluntary Service Overseas and other sending agencies.

Jean runs People Potential, which aims to help individuals and organisations to develop and use their potential in practical work through research, knowledge and training. People Potential runs courses in the UK and worldwide. Areas of work include APT, assistive furniture, educational toys, creative crafts and consultancies in helping small workshops to increase efficiency through batch production.

Over the years People Potential has developed links with people with disabilities and organisations in many parts of the world. It is now working with Source, an international information support centre based at UCL, and with Cerebral Palsy Africa (CPA).

For any advice or feedback please contact via the People Potential website, www.peoplepotential.org.uk, or the APT website, www.apbt.org.

Appendix B

Choosing appropriate play activities to engage a child's active involvement in therapy

CHILDREN need opportunities to play in order to learn. Young children play and learn in all their waking moments and, if we want to engage with them, we must understand the nature and purpose of their games.

At different stages in their development, children enjoy different play activities. The following table may help you to choose activities that the child you are working with is likely to enjoy.

Age	Activity
0–3 months	• Enjoys making eye contact with familiar people • Later, smiles in response to eye contact and smile from familiar person
3–5 months	• Enjoys being talked to. Enjoys songs • Likes to look at toys hanging within reach of his hands • Enjoys having toys placed in his hands. Learns to bat a toy with his hands • When placed prone he enjoys the sensation of scratching the floor with his fingers
6–11 months	• Laughs at peekaboo games. Likes to look at himself in a mirror • Recognises family members and know their names if told them often enough • Knows his own name • Manipulates all kinds of objects in his hands—brings everything to his mouth • Likes squeaky toys and rattles • Loves to be handled, carried about, bounced on his mother's lap or pushed along in a pushchair
12 months	• Enjoys hearing songs and nursery rhymes over and over again • Uses hands bilaterally: he can hold cup in one hand and drop object into it with the other or he can hold a large, light ball with two hands • Enjoys finding things that have been hidden • Enjoys picking up tiny things between his finger and thumb • Likes toys that he can pull and push along
18 months	• Imitates all kinds of sounds and actions. Loves to listen to his mother telling him what she is doing as she goes about her chores • Loves to fetch and carry familiar objects when asked • Enjoys putting things in containers and taking them out again • Likes to point to a few parts of his body that he knows • Enjoys looking at pictures of familiar objects

(continued)

(*continued*)

Age	Activity
2 years	• Likes climbing, swinging and sliding • Loves simple stories
3 years	• Enjoys playing with other children • Begins to enjoy pretending; pretends to drive the car or sweep the floor, for example • Loves to push himself about on a tricycle or pedal car • Loves stories with pictures

For a child with CP, who will find it difficult to do all these things for himself in a normal way, it is important for those working with him to help him so that he gains some of the experiences that will later help him to make sense of the world around him. For instance, it is important for a child to learn to reach out for toys and bat them with outstretched fingers before he learns to grasp and bring things to his mouth. It is important for a child to learn to hold a toy in two hands so that he can later learn to coordinate using his hands together. He can be helped to do these things by hand-over-hand assistance from those working with him. The experience will help him to try the activity by himself later.

USING PLAY DURING TREATMENT

Before planning a treatment session with a child, think about what it is you want to encourage the child to do and make sure the play activity does not do the opposite. For example, if you want to encourage a child to reach out while keeping her trunk upright and her head erect it may not be a good idea to offer her a toy that she will want to grasp and bring to her mouth, because this may cause her to use a total pattern of flexion. Instead, for example, you could arrange for a ball to be suspended on a string just above where the child will be lying in prone. Straight away she will try to reach up and push the ball away. She will then hold her head up to see the ball swing back.

If, in your treatment, you want to facilitate rotation in a child of about 2 who enjoys putting objects into a container, she will want to reach up with rotation from where she is sitting to where you are holding a small block. She can then bend down and drop it into a container which you have placed near her opposite knee. All the better if the container is a tin, because the brick will make a satisfying noise as it is dropped in.

Another variation on this game is to prop a plank with raised edges on a chair. The child uses two hands to lift an inflatable ball onto the higher end of the plank and watches it roll down to knock over the light plastic bottle you have placed in its path. This is a very useful game for a child to play while you are trying to facilitate active extension of her hips and knees. You may need to ask her mother to fetch the ball and replace the bottle each time, but you will be amazed at how many times the child will be willing to carry on playing this game. This is because the activity gives her the opportunity to practise and discover how to make things happen, and this is appropriate to her present level of play.

Often, working with children with athetosis, we want them to hold postures rather than to move. In this case it is important to find interesting things for the child to watch or pay attention to. Perhaps you want the child to hold her trunk steady in standing while you facilitate extension in her knees and weight-bearing on straight arms. You could try getting her mother to read her an interesting story, or you could get her to play peekaboo, or maybe she could watch another child rolling the ball down the plank.

Action songs that children do as a group are very interesting and exciting for children aged between 3 and 5 years. It is worthwhile trying to arrange for several children of similar ages and conditions to come for treatment together.

Glossary

ABDUCTION	Movement of a limb to the side away from the body.
ACETABULUM	Bony cup-shaped hollow in the pelvis that holds the head of the femur in the hip joint.
ACHILLES TENDON	Tendon at the back of the heel that connects the calf muscles to the heel bone (calcaneous).
AGONIST	Muscle or groups of muscles that carry out the primary action in a movement. For example, the elbow flexors are the agonists when the elbow is flexed against gravity.
ADDUCTION	Sideways movement of a limb from abduction back to the body or across the body.
ALIGNMENT	Three or more parts in a straight line.
ANTAGONIST	Muscle or group of muscles that pay out in a coordinated way to allow the agonists to carry out a smooth movement. For example, the elbow extensors are the antagonists when the elbow is flexed against gravity.
ANTERIOR	In front of.
ASSOCIATED MOVEMENT	Coordinated movements occurring in the *absence* of spasticity. They are seen during early childhood where movements are more in total patterns. They are also seen throughout life when new motor skills are being learnt or where there is effort. Examples include mirror movements and facial grimacing.
ASSOCIATED REACTION	Abnormal increase in tone in one part of the body as a result of effort in another which is less affected. The reaction is associated with spasticity and is seen as a movement in a child with mild to moderate spasticity and felt as an increase in tone in a child with severe spasticity.
ASYMMETRIC	One side of the body acts in a different way to the other.
ATAXIC, ATAXIA	Difficulty in coordinating movement—poor balance—and clumsy, awkward voluntary movements.
ATHETOID, ATHETOSIS	This term comes from a Greek word meaning 'of no fixed posture'. Children with athetoid CP have no fixed posture because of involuntary movements and lack of coordinated co-contraction.

BALANCE	Ability to stay in and regain a position when the influence of gravity would otherwise cause a fall. This ability is the result of the interaction of righting, equilibrium and protective reactions.
BASAL GANGLIA	Part of the brain.
BASE	The supporting part of the body. In standing, the base will be the feet; in sitting, the pelvis, thighs and perhaps feet.
BODY AXIS	An imaginary line drawn through the body from the middle of the head down to between the feet, when the person is in alignment.
BOTULINUM	Botulinum or botulin toxin (also known as botox or Dysport) is a very poisonous substance used in very minute doses to treat muscle spasm. It is injected with great care at the exact place where the nerve is attached to the spastic muscle. It then blocks the release of some of the chemical from the nerve that activates the muscle to contract.
BREAKING UP PATTERNS	Changing one or two elements of the stereotyped patterns of movement that children with spasticity try to use to function. For example, the stereotyped pattern of extension in the lower limb is adduction, inward rotation and some flexion at the hip, extension in the knee and plantarflexion at the ankle. The pattern could be broken up (and be more functional) by introducing either dorsiflexion at the ankle or extension in the hip (or both).
CALCANEOUS	Heel bone.
CALF MUSCLES	Muscles at the back of the lower leg that plantarflex the foot and flex the knee.
CALLIPERS	Metal or plastic and metal supports that hold either the ankle or the knee joint rigid.
CEREBELLUM	Part of the brain.
CENTRAL NERVOUS SYSTEM	The brain and spinal cord.
CO-CONTRACTION	Normal co-contraction is the simultaneous activation of agonist and antagonist to give mobility with stability. It provides us with normal postural tone and allows smooth graded co-ordinated movement.
CONTRACTION	Normal activity in a muscle that causes it to shorten and bring about movement in a joint.
CONTRACTURE	Permanent shortening of a muscle, muscle tendon or joint structure. Once a contracture becomes established, fibrous

tissue is laid down, and then it can only be lengthened by surgery.

COORDINATION   Smooth, efficient movement caused by the activity of muscles working together and controlled by the nervous system.

CORTEX   Part of the brain.

CREEPING   Moving around the floor in prone on elbows. Legs are mostly inactive.

CRAWLING   Moving around the floor on hands and knees.

DEFORMITY   Abnormal body posture or limb position. It can be fixed or unfixed.

DISSOCIATION   Ability to move one body part and keep the rest still or to move one limb in one direction while another moves in the opposite direction, e.g., in crawling.

DIPLEGIA   Whole body affected by CP but lower limbs more than upper limbs.

DISTAL, DISTALLY   Situated away from central part of body.

DORSAL SPINE   That part of the spine between the neck and the lower back.

DORSIFLEXION   Movement at ankle joint that brings heel down and toes up: standing on the heels.

ENCEPHALITIS   Inflammation of the brain caused by infection. It can cause lasting damage to the brain.

EPILEPSY   Sometimes called fits or seizures. It is abnormal electrical impulses in the brain causing involuntary muscle contractions. These can vary from very slight to severe spasms and unconsciousness.

EQUILIBRIUM   State of balance.

EQUILIBRIUM REACTIONS   Automatic and highly complex movements which serve to maintain and regain balance before, during and after displacement of the centre of gravity.

EVERSION   Turning the sole of the foot outwards away from the other foot.

EXTENSION   To 'extend' means to stretch out or make longer. Extension in the body means the limbs are straight the trunk is upright or stretched out and the head is up or pushed back.

EXTENSOR TONE   The state of tension in those muscles that extend the body.

FACILITATION   A handling technique to make active movement easier—or to make active movement possible where it was not possible before.

FEMUR   Long bone of the thigh.

FINE MOTOR CONTROL	Coordinated hand function, allowing such things as writing or tying shoe laces.
FLEXION	The opposite of extension. The limbs are bent up and the trunk is curved forward. In full flexion the body and limbs would be curled up into a ball.
FLEXOR TONE	The state of tension in those muscles that flex the body and limbs.
FUNCTION	Purposeful activity—useful motor abilities such as being able to hold one's head erect.
GRADING OF MOVEMENT	Smooth controlled movement.
GREATER TROCHANTER	Prominent bony part of femur which can be felt at the upper and outer part of the thigh.
HALF KNEELING	This is an upright kneeling position where weight is taken on one knee while the other leg is bent forward with the foot flat on the floor.
HAMSTRINGS	Large muscles at the back of the thigh that extend the hip joint and flex the knee.
HANDLING	The way in which we move or touch a child.
HEMIPLEGIA	Kind of CP where the whole of one side of the person's body is affected. It can be the right or the left side.
HYPEREXTENSION	Extends more than normal.
HYPERMOBILE	Abnormally wide range of movement in joints.
HYPERTONIA	Increased tone in muscles. Neural hypertonia is caused by damage to the central nervous system. Non-neural hypertonia is caused by local changes in muscles and joints. If hypertonus is constant, though changing in degree, the child is said to have spasticity.
HYPOTONIA	Low muscle tone.
INTERMITTENT SPASMS	These are often present in children with moderate spasticity or dystonic athetosis. They often occur in the abdominal muscles and can be uncomfortable or even painful, especially if they are associated with constipation. In dystonic children they can also produce strong extension of head and trunk with rotation to one side.
INWARD ROTATION	The turning inward of the whole arm or the whole leg. This movement can only take place at the hip or shoulder joint.
INVERSION	Turning the sole of the foot inwards towards the other foot.
INVOLUNTARY	Happens without the child wanting it to.

KEY POINTS OF CONTROL	These are parts of the body from where tone, postures and patterns of movement in other parts can be changed, controlled and guided.
LATERAL	Referring to the outer side of limbs.
LONG SITTING	Sitting on the floor with legs extended.
LUMBAR SPINE	Waist-level part of spine, above the pelvis and below the ribs.
MEDIAL	Referring to the inner side of limbs.
MENINGITIS	Inflammation of the outer covering of the brain due to an infection. It can cause lasting damage to the brain.
MOBILE WEIGHT-BEARING	Bearing weight on limbs or trunk while there is movement, either in the part which is bearing weight or in the rest of the body.
MORO REACTION	Seen in a very young normal baby: when the head falls back, the arms fly up and out and the fingers open. It is abnormal if it persists after about 5 months.
OPPOSITION OF THE THUMB	Movement of the thumb away from the fingers to allow grasp.
ORTHOSES, ORTHOTIC, ORTHOTISTS	Limb or trunk supports made of metal or plastic material. These are made by orthotists.
OUTWARD ROTATION	The turning outwards of the whole arm or the whole leg. This movement can only take place in the hip or shoulder joint.
OVERSHOOTING	Inaccurate targeting of a movement such as pointing to or reaching for an object.
PATELLA	Small bone on the point of the knee embedded in quadriceps muscle and unattached to any other bone.
PATHOLOGICAL	To do with abnormal signs.
PATTERNS OF MOVEMENT	When normal patterns of movement take place in a huge variety of ways to carry out everyday activities such as walking. *Abnormal patterns* are seen in a child with spasticity who can only move in a few stereotyped ways that are not functionally useful.
PELVIS	Bony framework that includes the pelvic bones and hip joints.
PLACENTA	Also called the after-birth, it is the structure that connects the unborn baby to the mother inside the uterus and provides nutrition and oxygen for the baby.
PLANTARFLEXION	Movement at the ankle joint when the toes are down and the heel up—standing on the toes.
POSTERIOR	Behind or at the back.

POSTURAL CONTROL	Ability to hold the body steady before, during and after a movement.
POSTURE	The position in which a person holds the body.
PRIMITIVE PATTERNS	Describes patterns of movement associated with a new-born baby.
PRONATION	Movement of the forearm that turns the palm downwards.
PRONE	Lying on the flexor surface of the body. The face can be down or turned to the side.
PROTECTIVE REACTIONS OR RESPONSES	Automatic movements that act to protect the body from injury, e.g., stretching out arms to protect face or taking a step to avoid falling.
PROXIMAL, PROXIMALLY	Close to central parts of the body.
PULL TO STAND	Before a young child can stand up from the floor alone he pulls himself up by holding on to the furniture or his mother. This is called pulling to stand.
QUADRIPLEGIA	Whole body affected.
QUADRICEPS MUSCLE	Muscle on the front of thigh that flexes the hip and extends the knee.
RECIPROCAL MOVEMENT	Complementary opposite movements as one leg moving forward and the other backwards during walking.
REFLEX	An automatic, involuntary response to a stimulus, e.g., knee jerk when the patellar tendon is tapped.
RIGHTING REACTION	These are automatic responses that work with equilibrium reactions to bring head and trunk back into alignment after activity.
ROTATION	Movement of one part of the body round the body axis. For example, a person rotates the trunk when they twist the top half of the body to one side, leaving the lower part of the body in a neutral position.
SACRUM	The bone at the base of the spine connecting the two sides of the pelvis.
SCAPULA	Wing-shaped bone that forms the back of the shoulder girdle and moves freely around the ribs in the upper back.
SELECTIVE MOVEMENT	Coordinated movement in one part of the body that does not influence other parts. For example, grasping an object without flexing the whole arm.
SHOULDER GIRDLE	The bony framework that includes the collar bone and the shoulder blade.
SIDE LYING	Lying on either the right or the left side.

SPASTICITY, SPASTIC	Abnormal stiffness in muscles that makes a child move in a limited, stereotyped way, or may even make movement impossible.
STARTLE RESPONSE	Child jumps, or lifts his head and arms, when there are loud noises or sudden movements.
STEREOTYPED	'Stereotyped' means always the same; no variety. Used to describe the abnormal patterns of movement associated with spasticity, it means, for example, that the child can only flex his arm with pronation and that when he extends his legs it is always with adduction.
STERNUM	The breast bone.
SUPINATION	Movement of the forearm that turns the palm of the hand upwards.
SUPINE	Lying on the extensor surface of the body. The face may be turned upward or to either side.
SYMMETRY	Both sides of the body are the same.
SYNAPSES	Connections between brain cells.
TENDON	The part of the muscle that connects it to a bone.
TONE	State of tension in muscles or state of readiness to become tense or move.
VENTRICLE	A ventricle is a part of the body filled with fluid. The four ventricles in the brain produce fluid that bathes and protects the brain and spinal cord.
VISUAL PERCEPTION	The brain's ability to interpret the messages sent from the eyes.
WINDSWEPT	This refers to the position of a child's legs when one leg is more abducted and outwardly rotated and the other is more adducted and inwardly rotated, making them look as though they have been blown sideways by the wind.

Index

abduction, 74, 160

acetabulum, 78, 79, 80

Achilles tendon, 74, 75–81, 83, 87

adaptive responses, 203

adduction, 33f, 45, 73, 99, 116, 136f, 146f, 154, 160, 189

agonists, 20, 52

Anderson, J., 177n

ankle foot orthoses (AFOs), 85

ankle joints, 85

antagonists, 20, 52

anxiety, 222

appropriate paper-based technology (APT), 22, 23, 155, 228–39

aspiration, silent, 208, 210

associated reactions, 65

asymmetry, of movements, 27

ataxia: 15, 42, 58, 91, 113–15
    benefits from weight-bearing, 149
    dressing/undressing of children with, 114
    features of, 56
    principles of treatment, 113
    and spasticity, 116, 117

athetoid cerebral palsy, children with: 59, 116, 117, 160
    benefits from weight-bearing, 149
    hypersensitivity in, 186
    rolling into prone, 68
    sensory processing problems in, 176
    and 'spasticity', 58
    walkers for, 165–66
    and walking, 42

athetosis, children with: 15, 58, 91
    postural control of, 116
    types of, 54

Ayres, Jean, 173–74

balance, and control, 14

balance reactions, 21, 25, 27, 34, 114

balanced model. *See* models of therapy/rehabilitation

basal ganglia, 15

basic tone, 60

bathing aids, 168–71

bean bags/sand bags, use in treatment, 184, 194, 195, 199

benches and stools, use in treatment, 145–47

Bhreathnach, Eadaoin, 177

biting patterns, 221

bite reflex, 207, 221–22

Blanche, E.I., 173n, 174n, 179

Bobath, Berta, 20

Bobath, Karel, 20

Bobath approach, 12, 20–21. *See also* neuro-developmental therapy

body mitt, use in treatment, 199

body temperature, 178

botulinum treatment, 20

'bow and arrow' posture, 64

brain:
    control and coordination of movement, 14
    sub-cortical area, 172, 173

brain stem sensory integration dysfunction, 173

bunny hopping, 40, 65

calf muscles:
    and flexing of the knees, 75
    lengthening ability of, 74

calcaneous, 85

callipers, 86

cerebellum, 15

cerebral palsy:
    assessing a child with, 25–49
    and associated problems, 16
    causes of, 17–18, 173
    characteristics of postural tone in, 15–16
    classification of, 50
    kinds of, 15
    mixed, children with, 116–17

modern definition of, 13–15
secondary effects of, 71
treatment for, 19
chairs:
    with curved back, 238–39
    making of, 228–37
    prone angle (forward-tilting), 157–58
    reclining, 155–56
    upright, and table, 156–57
    use in treatment, 153, 155–58
    See also appropriate paper-based technology
        (APT)
Chambers, Robert, 120
chewing of food, 185, 204, 205, 218–19, 222
chewing skills, 225
child/children with cerebral palsy:
    care of, in institutions, 193
    with disabilities, 10, 120
    lifting/handling of, 29, 133–37
    observation of, held in standing, 32–33
    people working with, 22–24
    personality characteristics of, 59
    positioning of:
        prone on the mat, 31–32
        sitting on the floor, 29–30
        sitting on stool, 29
        in supine, 89
    pre-term, 177, 194–95
    suggested positions for dressing, 138–40
    therapist's relationship with, 132–33
    tone, assessing, 72
choreo-athetosis, children with: 54–55, 104–12
    case study, 195–96
    experience of grasping, 107, 110
    lack of head and trunk control, 105
    treatment, 104
    trunk control, 111, 112
    walking, 111, 112
claw toes, 76, 83–85
co-contraction, 52, 115, 116
Coleridge, Peter, 122
community-based rehabilitation (CBR), 10, 121, 122
compensatory activities, 43
'compression':
    as proprioceptive input, 181
    through child's limbs, 105

computerised tomography (CT) scan, 17
constipation, water intake when in, 225
contractures: 13, 42
    assessment of, 72–76
    assistive devices:
        callipers, 86
        footwear, 85–86
        splints, 85
    prevention of, 85–86, 124
    surgery to treat, 86–87
    See also deformities
coping mechanism, of the family, 120
cortex, damage to, 15
cough reflex, 203
crouch gait, 82, 83
cruising, 42

deformities, 42, 65–66, 76–85. *See also* contractures
dental hygiene, 224
deep pressure, on joints, 176
DeGangi, G.A., 173n, 174n, 177n
diagnosis, 16–17, 50
diplegia, 42, 51, 77, 78, 88
dislocation, 112
dissociation, between legs, 41, 65
distal key point, 92
Doidy cup, 219
dorsal spine, 76
drinking:
    introduction of babies to, 204
    normal pattern of, 205–206
    oral stage, 205
    pre-oral stage, 205
    safe pattern of, 219–20
    swallow, 206
drugs for cerebral palsy, 19–20
dystonic athetosis, children with: 54, 56, 112–13, 160
    spasms in, 112, 113
    treatment for, 112

eating and drinking, difficulties in:
    developing chewing, 218–19
    hands, involvement of, 216
    management of, 212–20
    normal pattern of, 205–206
    oral control, 216–17
    positioning of child, 213–16
    spoon-feeding, 217–18

eating and drinking patterns, assessment of: 206–12
    communication at mealtimes, 211–12, 214
    gastro-oesophageal influx, 210–11
    jaw movement, 204, 207, 209, 212, 218
    lips, use in, 207, 210
    oral sensory awareness, 208–209
    oral stage, 209–10
    position of child, 206–207
    pre-oral stage, 206
    swallowing, 210–12
    tongue movement in, 207–208, 210
electrotherapy, 11
encephalitis, 16
epilepsy, 16
equipment, examples of useful: 199
    at treatment centres and at home, 141–71
    for trying out, 150–51
    for use at home, 152–71
exercise, 129
extension: 94, 99, 212
    coordination between flexion and, 21
    maintaining, 98
    treatment for, 96
extensor(s): 52
    abnormal pattern of, 62
    muscles, 190
    spasms, 113
    spasticity, 157
    thrust, 98

facial expression, 178
family(ies):
    concerns, and assessment, 58–59
    giving information to, by therapists, 123, 129
    therapist and, 123, 124–25
femur, 78, 79, 80, 81
fits, 16
flexion: 33, 43, 54, 94, 95, 153, 212
    abnormal pattern, 62
    coordination between, and extension, 21
flexor spasms, 222, 223
flexor spasticity:
    children with, 52, 91, 102, 115
    of legs, 116
floor mats, use in treatment, 141, 142
foot-straps, 160, 162

footwear, 85–86
fractures, 112
fundoplication, 211

gag reflex, 203
gait, 43
gastrostomy tube, feeding through, 226
grading, 20
grasping: 61
    by child with athetosis, 110
    sensori-motor experience of, 110
gravity/gravitational:
    influence of, 63, 64
    insecurity, 176, 197
groin straps, 156
gums, 224
gut, dysmotility of, 211

hammock, use in treatment, 196, 199
hamstring:
    assessing the length of, 74, 75
    contractures, 74
handling skills, 43–49, 91, 123, 130–31, 135–37
hands, involvement in eating, 216
Hari, Maria, 19
head:
    control, 204
    movement, reaction-related, 64
    and trunk, positioning of, while eating, 216
hearing, problem in, 16
heel cups, 160
hemiplegia: 42, 77, 101
    and associated reactions, 65
    and distal key point, 92, 93
    right-sided, 72, 73
hips:
    adduction of, 99
    dislocation of, 76, 80–81, 87
    extension, 150
    joint, assessing the stability of, 80
hot packs, 11
hyperbilirubinaemia, 18
hypersensitivity: 177, 179, 209
    hyposensitivity and, 175–76
    at mealtimes, 220
    reducing, 222
    touch, 192
    vestibular, 188–90

hypertonia: 15, 51, 114–17
    abnormal patterns associated with, 62
    child with changeable, 51
    child with severe, 51
    features of, 57
    principle of treatment of, 115
hypotonia:
    definition, 15, 51
    features of, 57, 58
    treatment of, 115–16
hyposensitivity: 177, 180, 209
    and hypersensitivity, 175–76
    at mealtimes, 221
    touch, 192–93
    vestibular, 186–88

iliac spine, 80
inserts, 162–63
internal rotation, of child's legs, 99
involuntary movements, 27

joint(s):
    alignment, 71
    compression, use of, 115
    dislocation, 87
    of knees, 81
    limitation, 73
    sub-laxated dislocated joints, 87

knee:
    hyperextension of the, 33, 76, 81, 82
    joints, 81
knee blocks, 157
kneeling, pull to standing from, 41
key points of control: 91–92, 117
    distal, 92
    proximal, 92
    use of, 92–94, 104
kyphosis, 76, 77, 78, 79

learning capacity, 120
learning difficulties, 16, 132
lips, use of while eating and drinking, 204–207, 210, 212
lordosis, 76, 78, 79
lycra band, use in treatment, 184, 199

magnetic resonance (MR) imaging, 17
malnourishment, 211
medical boots, 85
medical model. See models of therapy/rehabilitation
medical plinths (padded tables), use in treatment, 141, 142
Mendis, Padmani, 122
meningitis, 16
Mobility Opportunities Via Education (MOVE), 19
models of therapy/rehabilitation:
    balanced, 121
    medical, 121, 124
    social, 121
moderate spasticity:
    associated reactions, 101
    crawling, 101, 102
    flexor spasms in the hips, 102
    'moderate spastic diplegia': 58
        upright chair for children with, 157
    treatment, 100–104
    walking, 101
Moro reaction, 27, 28
mothers, participation in therapy, 148
motor:
    control, fine, 14, 69–70
    coordination, 208
    deficits, 174
    development, 38
    functions, achieving basic, 66–70
mouthing reactions, 178
movement activities: 27, 62
    abnormal patterns of, 27, 66
    disorder of, 13
    distally, 20
    normal, 21
    observation of, 178
    quality of, 27
    selective, 14
    sensation of, to the brain, 14, 15
    sensitivity to, 188
    sequences of, 48–49
Move International Curriculum, 19
muscles, 14
muslin cloth, use in treatment, 199

naso-gastric tube, feeding through, 226
neck:
    cushion, for treatment, 138f, 139f, 154f, 155–56
    elongation of the back of, 207, 225

flexion, 62*f*, 104
flexor spasticity of, 104
extension, 104, 207, 212
position of, in eating, 205, 207, 213, 215–16, 219*f*, 224
retraction, 62*f*, 96–97
nervous system, 173, 175
Neuro-Developmental Therapy (NDT), 12, 18, 20, 181
neuroplasticity, 21
nutritional issues, 225–26

occupational therapy (OT), therapists, 18, 196
oesophagitis, 223
oesophagus, 211
oral:
    control, 213, 214, 224
    hygiene, 224–26
    motor problems, 201
    sensory awareness, 208–10
    skills, 204

paralysis, of the brain, 13
patella (kneecap), 76, 81–82, 83
pelvic belt, 162
Peto, Andreas, 19
phenobarbitone, 16
physiotherapy, -therapists, 10, 18, 196
placenta, 18
plantarflexion: 33
    at ankle, 82
platform swing, therapeutic use of, 199
postural patterns: 14, 15, 61–65
    disorder of, 13
    and movement of the child, 61
postural tone: 15–16, 20, 44, 178, 206, 209
    abnormal, 17, 44
    assessment and treatment of, 45–46
    in prone, 47
    in sitting, 44–45
    in supine, 46–47
pregnancy:
    and causes of cerebral palsy, 17
    patterns of movement of child in, 14
prone standing frame, 222, 223
proprioceptive:
    activities, 179, 180, 181, 186
    information, 194
    sensation, 174, 195

protective responses: 27, 203
    coughing, 203
    gagging, 203
proximal:
    fixation, 20, 111
    key point, 92
    sensation, 175
pushchairs, inserts in, 162, 163
PVC pipes, use in bathing, 169–70

quadriceps muscle, 81
quadriplegia: 42, 51, 77, 78
    moderate, 89
    spastic, 25

reflexes, 14
reflux, gastro-oesophageal, 201, 206, 210–11, 212, 222–23
Reilly, S., 201
rocker bottom feet, 76, 82–83, 84
rollator, use in walking, 150
rolls, use in treatment, 143–44, 182, 185, 199
rooting reflex, 203

saliva production, while eating, 208
'sandwich sitting', 147
scapula, 76
scoliosis, 76, 77
scooter board, use in treatment, 199
sensation:
    and motor coordination, 208–209
    difficulty in processing, 16
    managing problems of, 220–21
sensori-motor experience, 114, 172
sensory:
    awareness, abnormal, 209
    information, 172, 173, 175
    integration, theory of, 173–75
    integration problems:
        assessing, 178–80
        treatment for, 181–93
    modulation difficulty, 176
    processing dysfunction: 176–77, 178
        athetoid cerebral palsy, 176
        in children born pre-term, 177
        spasticity, 176–77
    responses, 175
'shut down', 181, 191

'sequence of movement', 34–43
shoulder:
    and elbow dislocation, 76, 85
    girdle, 76
    straps, 162
shower aids. *See* bathing aids
shuffling, bottom-shuffling, 40
side-lying board, 154–55
sitting balance, 168–69
sitting up: 38
    support needed, 26–27
sleeping difficulties, 194
social model. *See* models of therapy/rehabilitation
spasms: 206
    in children with dystoxic athetosis, 112–13
    intermittent, 47
spastic diplegia:
    case study, 196–97
    and use of proximal key point, 92, 93
    and walking, 65
spastic quadriplegia, 66–67, 87
spasticity: 13, 15, 25
    and difficulty with bilateral integration, 176
    moderate, features of, 53
    and motor planning, 176
    pattern of, 64
    and poor body awareness, 176
    and sensory processing problems, 176–77
    severe:
        features of, 51–53
        feeding a child with, 96, 98
        treatment of, 94–100
    transitory, 57
speech and language therapists, 12, 18
spinal cord, 14, 77
splint(s):
    gaiter, 151
    how to make, 151
    use in treatment, 85, 151
spoon-feeding, 217–18, 221
standing, in children with spasticity: 42
    pull to, from all-four kneeling, 41
    pull to, from sitting on a stool, 41–42
standing frames: 158–61
    benefits of, 153
    placing the child in, 161–62
    prone angle, 158–59

supine standers, 158, 159
    upright, 158, 161, 162
    use in treatment, 150
standing tables:
    electrically operated, 147
    use in treatment, 147–48
startle response, 27
sternum, 217
stimulation:
    tolerance of, 106
    use of, 115
subluxation: 87
    of the hip, 76, 78–80
suck–swallow response, 203
supination, 76, 110
synapses, 21

tactile:
    activities, 179, 180, 181
    processing, activity ideas to improve, 192–93
    sensations, in children with spasticity, 177
    sensory input, 191
    sensory problem, 198
    system, 174
'tapping' technique: 181
tendons, 14
therapy: 18–19
    ball, use of, 182, 184, 186, 187, 190, 197, 199
    centres, 21
    play activities in, 240–42
thumb, opposing, 76
toilet chairs, 166–68
tone:
    bent, 83
    extensor, 45, 89, 180
    flexor, 89
    fluctuating, 51, 57, 77
    high, 56, 72, 102, 115, 212
    intermittent, 51, 56
    low, 27, 45, 57–58, 69–70, 72, 76, 81, 115, 151, 155, 156
    making the, more normal, 89–94
    See also postural tone
tone influencing patterns (TIPs), 89, 101, 104, 117
tongue movement, while eating, 205–208, 210, 212, 224

tongue thrust, 207, 221
tooth and gum problems, 224–25
toys, use in treatment, 151–52, 199
tricycles, 164
trochanter, greater, 80
trunk:
    control:
        and athetoid child, 111, 112
        children with poor, 157
        reducing spasticity in the, 98
        rotation, introducing, 190
    extension and rotation of, 146
tumour, 17

ultrasound, 17

V-shaped pillow, use in treatment, 182, 185, 199
ventricles, 18
vestibular:
    activities, 179, 180, 181, 186
    hypersensitivity, 188–90
    hyposensitivity, 186–88
    processing, activities to improve, 186–90
    receptors, 174

sense, 174
system, 174
visual perception, 18
Vojta, Vaclav, 19
Vojta reflex locomotion, 19

walk/walking:
    aid, use in treatment, 148–50
    children learning to, 42–43
    wheelbarrow, 114, 115
walkers:
    baby, 163, 164
    wheeled, 165–66
weaning, 203
wedges, 144–45, 153–54
weight-bearing: 91, 103, 105, 139
    mobile, 38–39, 70, 90, 91*f*, 92*f*, 102, 113, 148–49, 181
wheelchairs, 162
wobble board, use in treatment, 199
wooden horse, 164
World Health Organization (WHO), 121
W-sitting, 30, 54, 55*f*, 94, 158

About the author

Archie Hinchcliffe is a Consultant Physiotherapy Trainer specialising in training therapists and community workers working with children in developing countries. She co-leads a biennial short course at the Bobath Centre in London specifically targeted at therapists intending to work in developing countries, and is a Trustee of Cerebral Palsy Africa, a Scottish charity founded in 2005 to support training programmes for therapists and others working with children with cerebral palsy in African countries.

Archie Hinchcliffe has extensive hands-on experience of working with children with cerebral palsy in many countries in the Middle East and Africa. She lives in Hutton, near Berwick-upon-Tweed in the UK.